TREATING SEX OFFENDERS IN CORRECTIONAL INSTITUTIONS AND OUTPATIENT CLINICS: A GUIDE TO CLINICAL PRACTICE
William E. Prendergast, PhD

SOME ADVANCE REVIEWS

"Fascinating, riveting, shocking, frightening, but also hopeful. If you want to understand what rapists, child molesters, and incest perpetrators are like, how they became so violence-prone, how important this developmental background is to their rehabilitation, how they can be treated and returned to society as productive citizens, and what characteristics and training one needs to help such individuals, Prendergast covers all these issues in this unique, realistic, and extremely useful book."

Robert T. Francoeur, PhD, ACS
Fairleigh Dickinson University
Madison, NJ

"This is a stunningly practical book, not only for clinicians, but for offenders, victims, and the parents of those who have been sexually abused. Dr. Prendergast's thirty years of research and development outline steps that can be implemented by everybody concerned with the field."

Vera Diamond
Executive Director
Breakthrough Training Programmes in the Field
of Childhood Sexual Abuse, London

Treating Sex Offenders in Correctional Institutions and Outpatient Clinics

A Guide to Clinical Practice

HAWORTH Criminal Justice,
Forensic Behavioral Sciences
& Offender Rehabilitation

Nathaniel J. Pallone, PhD
Senior Editor

New, Recent, and Forthcoming Titles:

Treating Sex Offenders in Correctional Institutions and Outpatient Clinics: A Guide to Clinical Practice by William E. Prendergast

Comparative Perspectives on Police by Dilip K. Das

Treating Sex Offenders in Correctional Institutions and Outpatient Clinics

A Guide to Clinical Practice

William E. Prendergast, PhD

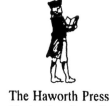

The Haworth Press
New York • London • Sydney

The Haworth Press, Inc., 10 Alice Street, Binghamton, NY 13904-1580
EUROSPAN/The Haworth Press, 3 Henrietta Street, London WC2E 8LU England
ASTAM/The Haworth Press, 162-168 Parramatta Road, Stanmore (Sydney), N.S.W. 2048 Australia

Library of Congress Cataloging-in-Publication Data

Prendergast, William E.
    Treating sex offenders in correctional institutions and outpatient clinics: a guide to clinical practice / William E. Prendergast.
      p.   cm.
    Includes bibliographical references and index.
    ISBN 1-56024-206-X (alk. paper). — ISBN 1-56024-207-8 (pbk.)
    1. Sex offenders — Rehabilitation. 2. Psychosexual disorders — Treatment. I. Title.
HV9276.P74 1991
365.6'6 — dc20
                                                                     91-24024
                                                                          CIP

This book is dedicated to the late RALPH BRANCALE, M.D., *who was my original mentor and pushed me into the field;* MY WIFE, MILDRED, *who supported and tolerated me through the worst of times and who provided very, very direct aid in the preparation of this manuscript;* MY SON, SHAWN, *who was my constant support on both a technical and personal basis and who never let me quit, especially when the computer intimidated me;* NATHANIEL J. PALLONE, Ph.D., *of Rutgers University, who became an unexpected and wonderful mentor and friend; to my colleagues and co-workers over the course of the years at Rahway Treatment Unit and at the Adult Diagnostic & Treatment Center, Avenel, of the New Jersey Department of Corrections, who contributed to the development and refinement of the ideas expressed in this manuscript; and to the thousands of sex-offenders and survivors of sexual abuse who taught me everything I know today.*

Contents

About the Author

WILLIAM E. PRENDERGAST served as Director of Professional Services at the Adult Diagnostic & Treatment Center in Avenel, a specialized unit of the Department of Corrections of the State of New Jersey statutorily charged with the diagnosis and treatment of repetitive, habitual, or compulsive sex offenders from the Center's opening in 1976 to his retirement in 1991. Prior to that appointment, Prendergast had served for nine years as Director of the Rahway Treatment Unit housed at Rahway State Prison, the predecessor to ADTC, and as a staff clinical psychologist at the New Jersey State Diagnostic Center at Menlo Park. Prendergast is presently engaged in lecturing, teaching, and training of sex therapists and correctional psychologists, social workers, and administrators and also maintains a limited private practice in sex therapy.

A native of Connecticut, Prendergast was educated at Fairfield University and the University of Detroit and received his Ph.D. from Walden University. He is certified as a sex therapist by the American Association of Sex Educators, Counselors, and Therapists (AASECT) and holds the Diplomate as Certified Sex Therapist and Clinical Supervisor of the American Board of Sexology. In 1991, he was presented the Distinguished Service Award of the New Jersey Child Assault Prevention Project for his contributions to treatment and the training of other professionals in the specialized techniques of treating sex offenders in correctional institutions and outpatient clinics.

Preface

During my thirty years of working with both sex offenders and their victims, it has become all too apparent that traditional treatment concepts, methodologies and frameworks *do not always work.*

We opened the first sex offender treatment facility in New Jersey on May 15, 1967 with only myself and a secretary as staff. One hundred (100) sex offenders were then transferred from the three (3) state mental hospitals and other correctional facilities where they had been housed since the Sex Offender Statute first was enacted in 1949. For more than a year, psychologists, psychiatric social workers and psychiatrists fumbled around, attempting to treat our first group of offenders with traditional methods. All forms of then-known therapy modalities including traditional, individual and group techniques were tried with little success. *Nothing seemed to work!*

The literature of the time offered little help. It became apparent that if the program were to succeed, new methods were needed to meet the needs of this very distinct group of individuals.

At the end of that first calendar year, a meeting was held with the then five or six (5 or 6) per-diem consultants (clinical psychologists and psychiatric social workers). There was an immediate consensus that what we were trying to do was not working. It was obvious that all of the treatment staff including its director, the consultants, and even the offenders, themselves, were frustrated.

During this period, several schools of psychotherapy were represented: Freudians, Behaviorists, Gestalt Psychologists Rogerians and eclectics. However, none of the staff felt that they were meeting the needs of this unique population.

Following the philosophy of *"Anna"* in the King of Siam story: "By your pupils you'll be taught", a meeting was held in the one-room dormitory with the director (with no other staff present) and the then one-hundred (100) convicted repetitive compulsive sex offenders. In a totally open manner, the frustrations of the staff were discussed and the resident population was told that since they were the offenders and had the psychological and sexual problems that we needed their help.

As radical as this approach appeared, it was necessary since there were few other states treating sex offenders at the time where we could go for assistance. The available literature was void of any help except for a few works that did not apply.

A resident committee was formed to act as liaison and advisor to the staff. Almost immediately, suggestions and criticisms came pouring into the director's office, both critical and positive. As suspected, the offenders knew where their deficits were. They clearly listed needs that they felt were paramount in their treatment and gave the staff a totally new perspective. This feedback from the offenders worked so well that, from that day forward, a resident committee has been an integral part of the treatment program.

The second attempt at a solution consisted of a staff meeting at the director's home. I had always suspected that *there were certain traits that all the sex offenders had in common, despite the offense they had committed.* At this time we had a full variety of offenders in the unit: rapists, child- molesters (both pedophiles and hebophiles), incestuous fathers, and exhibitionists (*"flashers"*).

Regardless of professional background, the entire staff agreed that they had felt the same frustration during their contacts with the sex offenders in the last·year or more, preceding the meeting.

As a result of both attempts, the following principles and concepts for treatment emerged:

The *first* factor that became apparent was that *passive, non-directive or Rogerian techniques would not work, for us.* With a completely supportive environment, these individuals became comfortable but also remained totally blocked by defense mechanisms. This was due to their overwhelming need for acceptance and concomitant fear of rejection from the therapists (now perceived as parental substitutes).

A combination of *confrontation and supportive techniques* became the norm and worked. Each technique will be discuss later.

The *second* factor that became apparent, from meetings and discussions with the resident committee was that *homogenizing groups was a fatal error.* A group of all rapists, for example, became supportive of each other and teamed against the therapist. The agreement between group members was: "You protect me and I'll protect you."

Challenge and/or confrontation thus became neutralized in a ten to one (10-1) battle, where the therapist always lost.

In a group of all child-molesters, boredom and lack of participation or involvement became the major problem. The inherent passivity and paralyzing fears of this group made therapeutic interaction almost impossible.

Thus, the second principle of treating this specific population became to *mix all of the groups* with rapists, child molesters, incestuous fathers and "flashers" (the four main groups in the facility).

The *third* and next most important factor that we quickly learned was *not to believe anything that these individuals verbalized unless it was proven by behavior.*

As director, a challenge to the staff was made to: *name a single therapeutic change that could not be observed in the daily behavior of our residents.* To this day, no one has been able to name one specific example to dispute this maxim. This does not mean that the behavioral change must be seen in the therapeutic process alone. Evidence of any meaningful change will also occur in the individual's work, recreation, leisure time activities and in all of his interpersonal interactions. Therefore, work supervisors, teachers, correction officers and families, all were solicited for *changes* that they either did or did not observe in their connected-offender. No clues as to what we were looking for were ever given, only a generic inquiry as to how an individual was doing at the time.

The *fourth* factor became that *individual therapy, as the primary or exclusive treatment modality, did not work.* Since we considered the sex offender pathology a *peer* or adolescent crisis reaction phenomena (see Chapter 2), it was important that each offender expose himself and his problems to his peer group. It appeared that these individuals could easily *confess* their pathology, deviant thinking and behavior to a therapist since they saw the therapist as more of a *"father confessor"* who would accept anything they said, would not be punitive and would not criticize or reject them. Since they had a strong adolescent need for peer acceptance, *group* was considered the appropriate treatment milieu.

Also, the groups were needed to confirm/deny what the elusive, defensive and denying offender was saying. Living with each other, they knew things that it was impossible for the therapist to know that were essential to the treatment process. Thus the therapists were trained to use their groups to be sure that what was being portrayed by the *"man on the floor"* was real and not a manipulation or defensive response. This process became known as: *confirmation. Group therapy,* then, *became the treatment modality of choice* for this population.

The *fifth* principle that became quickly apparent was that *psychotherapy by itself would not work.* The pathology of the compulsive sex offender appeared to involve his entire being: body and mind, social nature and emotional being as well. Thus a *Holistic* or *Whole-Person* approach was adopted that will be discussed in Chapter 15 in some detail.

We now had a beginning and all of the therapists felt more comfortable treating this very individualistic and unique group of individuals.

In a similar way, we continued to learn, step-by-step, and after a period of a year or two began to feel that we were finally reaching this population and seeing proof of therapeutic change.

Today, from an original population of one hundred offenders, there are more than four hundred and sixty five in treatment (as of this writing) with thirteen (13) psychologists.

For the last thirty years of treating both the sex offender and the victim, I have also tried to share what I have learned and the mistakes that I have made through training seminars with many groups in New Jersey, in many other states around the country, and in the United Kingdom, as well. Participants have ranged from the general public, to parents of either offenders or survivors, to professionals of all types: medical doctors, registered nurses, psychiatrists and psychologists, and social workers, to survivors and even to sex offenders themselves.

The present work parallels workshops and courses that I conduct and may not be as *scholarly* as some would prefer. The language level is set for all of the audiences listed above, as much as possible. A parallel work on *the survivor* of sexual abuse, entitled: "The Merry-Go-Round-of-Sexual-Abuse" is in preparation as a continuation of this first work.

In the following chapters, each individual aspect of the makeup and treatment of the compulsive sex offender (as I have experienced them), whether in a residential setting or in my private practice, will be explored. For each of the many treatment techniques, its inception, the principles behind the technique and its evolution, as the population changed, will be discussed.

It is the author's hope that by sharing the fumbling and errors that were made early in our experience, we can prevent other therapists from making the same errors. This applies especially in using techniques or principles that were tried in our years of immersion in this field and that failed. To this end, this work is dedicated.

It should be noted that, in keeping with the Human Subjects Regulations of the Federal Government, while all of the case histories cited are based on real people, there have been sufficient changes made in age, race, nationality, employment, family-makeup, etc. to protect their identity. I have personally worked with each of the individuals discussed in some therapeutic modality or as their primary therapist.

William E. Prendergast

1

Distinguishing Characteristics of Sex Offenders: The *Who* of Treatment

It may be self-evident that, before treatment of a sex offender can begin, the therapist must know something of the *who* (that is, the characteristics of the disorder which the client or patient is suffering) and the *why* (that is, the motives the client or patient has in seeking treatment, whether treatment has been imposed or mandated by external bodies like courts or the criminal justice system, etc.) of the patient.

Yet is has been my experience that members of diverse professional groups (whether psychologists, social workers, mental health center workers, probation or parole officers) often know little about the *who* of the sex offender. In contrast, they may know much more about the *what* (that is, that the disorder to be treated is either a psychiatric disorder in sexual functioning or an illegal behavior, or both) and the *why* (usually because of court proceedings, or, less often, because the client has recognized unwanted thoughts or feelings that he or she fears may lead to illegal behavior).

As a result, the client may become a guinea pig for the therapist who is just beginning to work with sex offenders. The invariable result is frustration for both at best — or, in a worst-case scenario, more sex crimes and more victims.

To gauge the extent to which beliefs, especially those of beginning mental health workers, rest on myth or on fact, I often give a brief, unannounced self-scoring test at the beginning of a training workshop. Rarely is a hand raised indicating a score above 70%. That test is reproduced here. Take it yourself; then try to find the answers to the questions throughout the rest of the book or turn to the Appendix for the answers.

A CLINICALLY DERIVED TABLE OF TRAITS

When we began this work in May of 1967, as detailed in the preface, little was known empirically about the population that we had been assigned to treat. The entire staff agreed that we desperately needed some form of schematic picture of the characteristics of personality and behavior that have been found clinically and empirically to uniquely differentiate the sex offender.

Let us consider the importance of such a list. Our hypothesis was that *if* such a list could be constructed and could identify at least the principal characteristics of those offenders who have been convicted of criminal sexual behavior, *then* we would have the outline for an effective and comprehensive treatment program for this population. The list would enable us to choose treatment modalities to address traits, counteract deficits, and engender appropriate values and skills — or substitute effective skills for those which have proven ineffective or harmful [*Note 1*].

Each of these traits has been found in differing degree, and in differing combinations, in several thousands of cases that I have treated and/or examined diagnostically. While it is my personal belief, based on my own clinical experience and the insights my colleagues have shared with me, that each of these traits can be found in each sex offender, each trait may not always be immediately visible. Sex offenders are often clever, highly manipulative individuals with the strongest defense mechanisms that a

• BELIEFS ABOUT SEX OFFENDERS: MYTH OR REALITY?

Respond True or False. Find the answers as you read the following chapters — or, if you can't wait, skip ahead to Appendix I. Give yourself 10 points for each correct response.

☐ *1. All sex offenders, regardless of offense, have major personality traits in common.*

☐ *2. All sex offenders were themselves sexually victimized as children and this explains their behavior.*

☐ *3. Sex offender pathology can be genetically linked.*

☐ *4. Pedophiles and hebophiles have the same characteristics and prognoses for treatment success.*

☐ *5. Fixated pedophiles may appear normal in their social, work, and interpersonal functions.*

☐ *6. Hebophiles and incestuous fathers have many traits in common and a similar (and more positive) prognosis for treatment success.*

☐ *7. The King-of-the-Castle syndrome is a major distinguishing characteristic of incestuous fathers.*

☐ *8. Supportive and non-confrontational treatment techniques work better with sex offenders than other treatment modalities.*

☐ *9. Psychotherapy itself will produce positive results with sex offenders.*

☐ *10. Following their victimization, victims of sexual abuse have many traits in common with sex offenders.*

clinician may ever encounter (except, perhaps, for the true multiple personality). Therefore, a thorough understanding of interviewing techniques, specialized treatment techniques and many, many other caveats are necessary to work with this population.

Additionally, an understanding of the origin of each of these characteristics and the degree to which they control and deter-

- **A TABLE OF DISTINCTIVE CHARACTERISTICS OF SEX OFFENDERS**
  - ☐ *BASIC INADEQUATE PERSONALITY*
  - ☐ *NEGATIVE SELF-IMAGE (EXAGGERATED)*
  - ☐ *SELECTIVE PERCEPTION*
  - ☐ *EXAGGERATED CONTROL NEEDS*
  - ☐ *PERVASIVE GUILT-SUBJECTIVE JUDGMENT*
  - ☐ *NONASSERTIVE*
  - ☐ *POOR TO NO INTERPERSONAL RELATIONS*
  - ☐ *NO PEER INTERACTION*
  - ☐ *EMOTIONS SUPPRESSED/DISPLACED*
  - ☐ *STRONG SEXUAL PERFORMANCE NEEDS*
  - ☐ *SMALL PENIS COMPLEX (UNREAL)*
  - ☐ *DISTORTED SEXUAL VALUES*
  - ☐ *DEVIANT AROUSAL PATTERNS*
  - ☐ *DEFECTIVE GOAL-SETTING SYSTEM*
  - ☐ *EASILY DISCOURAGED — QUITS*
  - ☐ *IDENTITY CONFUSION*
  - ☐ *CLEVERNESS IN DEALING WITH OTHERS*
  - ☐ *HIGHLY MANIPULATIVE*

mine the lifestyles and behavioral repertoire of the offender is essential before treating the sex offender is possible. Each characteristic, along with its source and its importance and implications in treatment, will be discussed in detail in succeeding chapters.

The Obsessive Compulsive Pattern

It is not uncommon that, by the time he or she is apprehended and enters the criminal justice system, the sex offender has been committing deviate sexual acts for many years. In fact, a significant percentage of sex offenders began their deviant fantasies and behaviors in their late childhood or early adolescent years. What occurs strongly resembles an obsessive-compulsive disorder. In this disorder, compulsive and repetitive acts are preceded or accompanied by obsessive thoughts.

The distinguished encyclopedist of mental health Benjamin Wolman [1989, p. 236] defines *obsession* as:

> An idea or impulse which persistently preoccupies an individual even though the individual prefers to be rid of it. Obsessions are usually associated with anxiety or fear and may constitute a minimal or a major disturbance of or interference with normal functioning and thinking.

Similarly, Wolman [Ibid., p. 68] defines *compulsion* as:

> The state in which the person feels forced to behave against his or her own conscious wishes and judgment.

To clarify the above definitions, it may be easier to understand the process in the following manner:

- First, the idea occurs, usually triggered by some traumatic event. A fantasy quickly follows.
- The idea/fantasy persists, regardless of all attempts to eradicate or extinguish the idea. Obsession now exists.
- The obsession results in a masturbation fantasy to the deviant idea and becomes habitual, then compulsive. Here again, all attempts to eradicate or extinguish the fantasy fail.
- Over a period of time or physical development in the case of pre-adolescents, the masturbation no longer satisfies the obsession and the fantasy is then acted out in some form.
- In young to pre-adolescent children, the first form the obsession may take is either voyeurism or exhibitionism with the primary obsession in the fantasy during the act. While a ten to twelve year old may not have the strength or courage to commit an overt sexual act with someone, he can peep through a window to watch a woman undress or to watch a couple engage in intercourse. He masturbates as he imagines being in the room and being the actor in the event.
- As both his physical strength and body development increase, the behavior becomes more and more in tune with the *need* generated to complete the obsessive fantasy. At this point, the sex offender is the most dangerous and, if not detected, will victimize someone.

THE QUESTION OF CHOICE

While a disturbed childhood, poor parental relationships and sexual trauma help to explain the development of the sex offender and his choice of pathological behavior, it neither justifies nor exculpates that behavior. However unpopular such a concept may be among those of my colleagues (and perhaps particularly among my academic colleagues) who hew to a deterministic explanation of behavior, I believe strongly that free will still exists in these individuals, although it may be dimmed (but not eliminated) by the dynamics which lead to compulsive behavior. Shorn of the niceties that surround what the courts and the legislature have defined as the acceptable grounds for exculpation on the basis of psychological factors (that is, for a successful plea of not guilty by reason of insanity), this position essentially comports with the state of the law as well.

In the thousands of cases we have treated over the last three decades, each has demonstrated this principle. If offenders are asked to describe in minute detail the events immediately preceding the offense, there are always many, many points at which they could have altered their course of action. Some general examples may clarify the point.

Sexually assaultive persons (rapists, assaultive child molesters, forceful incestuous fathers) usually describe several points, from the inception of the urge to the completed act, at which they became afraid, had doubts, or considered stopping the scenarios. Many sexually assaultive persons admit to instances of a rape-in-progress where once the victim was subdued, on the ground and exposed, their need was satisfied and they left. Many seductive child molesters describe getting the child into the location of the act (a closet in the school, their apartment, etc.), undressing the child and then panicking and ending the intended molestation.

It is not difficult, during intensive-confrontive therapy, to elicit these conscious, mental interruptions of an intended sex crime scenario. The overwhelming evidence of all therapists we have dealt with supports the fact of the sex offender's ability to stop himself during the offense at several distinct points in the chronology of the crime, especially during the early phases of the compulsion.

This same *free-will-choice* exists in their masturbation fantasies; a majority of them reporting that they have interrupted a deviant fantasy and either changed the fantasy to something positive or stopped the masturbatory behavior completely. Unless we are dealing with overt psychosis, this appears to be a valid observation.

Then why doesn't this prevent sex crime?

Considering the depressed, quitting quality of the offender's personality, the answer appears simple and obvious. At the juncture of the event, when the doubt or *choice* occurs, their thought processes include:

- "Well, you've gone this far, you may as well finish it."
- "It's no worse to finish than to stop. The punishment will be the same."
- "I've already committed the sin, so I may as well get the pleasure."
- "If I finish it and make them feel good maybe they won't report me."
- "You know you're a pervert (rapist, child molester, etc.) so you may as well act like one."

The variety of justifications to continue the deviant fantasy/behavior is as strong as the variety of the reasons to interrupt or stop the behavior.

As we will see in the chapters on treatment, as treatment progresses and the offender becomes stronger and more positive toward himself, these interruptions become more frequent and more successful with the goal of extinction or, at least, substitution of normal behavior for the deviant behavior. It is not uncommon for sex offenders to report promises, desperate attempts that fail and many other means of attempting to extinguish the compulsion but it never works unless therapeutic intervention and sometimes removal from society (where the trigger-stimuli are) is accomplished. This is most true of the child-molester groups.

At this point an example is needed for clarification:

☐ ROB, *at age 29, is an obscene phone caller to older women who sound motherly. He asks them if they would allow him to perform sexual intercourse on them (using street-slang). From his earliest memories, Rob had problems with interpersonal relationships, especially with females. Rob was a fat little boy and not particularly good-looking, which did not help his relational problems. His mother was overprotective, seductive and had a strong to violent temper. Arguments and fights were frequent in his home. When Rob was 15 his parents separated and he moved to California with his mother. Within a month of their moving into their new home, Rob's mother moved him into her bedroom and into her bed, telling him that now he was the man in her life. She then proceeded to undress, fondle and fellate him, his first sexual experience outside of masturbation. These sexual encounters continued for several years, even when Rob finally found a girlfriend, whom the mother despised. Rob's mother never permitted him to have penetrating intercourse with her, stating: "You're not man enough or big enough to satisfy me that way. When you grow, I'll think about it!" The more Rob persisted, the more vehement were the refusals and rejections.*

Rob finally ran away and returned to the live with his father in the East and to work at his father's business where he was maltreated and verbally abused. No matter what he did, nothing satisfied his father, a demanding old-world type and a craftsman. Within a month, during which he compulsively masturbated to having intercourse with his mother, the obscene phone calls began. Fewer than 20 calls were made when he was apprehended by accident when he phoned a senator's wife, whose line was tapped due to threats against the senator's life. Rob was arrested and sent to my practice for treatment as a mandated condition of probation.

While his treatment will be discussed later in the training, some of his statements are relevant to this discussion:

- "No matter how hard I tried, I couldn't get having sex with my mother out of my mind."

- "Even if I masturbated to pornography or to the fantasy of my girlfriend with whom I am having sex, eventually my mother replaces all images in the act. If she doesn't I am unable to reach a climax."

- "I was always afraid my friends would find out and I knew it was abnormal but no matter how hard I tried the thoughts and fantasies as well as the masturbation became more frequent and more demanding. I even masturbated in the bathroom after just having an hour or more of sex with my mother, especially when she wouldn't let me fuck her."

- "At times, I thought that the only way to stop these things from happening was to kill myself and I even tried once but chickened out."

Guilt, sin, and fear of exposure, arrest, and imprisonment are all tried by the compulsive sex offender, to no avail. It is my belief, based on my clinical experience and that of many of my colleagues, that until the early sexual traumas are relived, ventilated and all the emotions and distorted values dealt with through therapy, no lasting or meaningful change will occur [*Note 2*]. Additionally, *the* harder the sex offender tries to stop his deviant thoughts, fantasies or behaviors, the stronger the compulsion becomes and the more frequently it occurs. Throughout our training and discussions, *compulsion* will always be understood as a characteristic of all sex offenders, and especially of the fixated-pedophile group.

NOTES

1. Optimally, such a list should extend to all sex offenders, regardless of their individual form of deviant behavior or their choice of victim by sex or age. As stated in the preface's chronology for the opening of the first treatment program in the state of New Jersey, after a year of fumbling around and trying all then-know treatment techniques, the entire staff felt quite strongly that regardless of the deviant behavior or offense, most of the offenders sent by the courts for treatment had certain identifiable traits in common. Each staff member, independently and without cross-discussion, was asked to submit a list of the major personality traits that he (women therapists were not permitted to be employed in the prison at that time) felt characterized the personality of the sex offender. Once the lists were tabulated, a meeting was held and the final list was developed. Next, using the list, the director and the staff reformulated the entire treatment program and developed modalities to deal with each of the delineated traits.

    The list fulfilled our expectations beyond our anticipation or hope, and, for the first time, the staff (as well as the patients) saw therapeutic progress begin. Changes in behavior, attitude and motivation were all observed both in and outside of the treatment unit (by officers, supervisors, families, etc.) and, over the next year or two, more and more treatment modalities were included in the program in accordance with the table, which became a base for the treatment program. While it was constructed in 1969, it is still is use and effective today.

2. Other experts in the treatment of sex offenders feel, to the contrary, quite strongly that aversive behavior therapy produces significantly more positive results. The reader is referred to the instructive volume *Rehabilitating Criminal Sexual Psychopaths: Legislative Mandates, Clinical Quandaries* by Dr. Nathaniel J. Pallone (Transaction Books, 1990). Pallone presents an excellent survey of both standard and aggressive methods of treatment for sex offenders and their legal constraints that includes such aggressive treatment modalities as bioimpedance measures, including surgical and chemical castration, and aversive modalities, including aversive behavior therapy, revulsion, electroshock, and

pharmacologically induced aversion (nausea). Examples and studies are included for each type of therapy.

2

The Inadequate Personality

Of all the traits that sex offenders have in common, none is as dominant and recurrent as that of the *inadequate personality,* a characteristic that is seen in each and every one of them.

Traditionally, *inadequate personality* has referred to:

That class of personality disturbances in which the individuals are characterized by inadaptability, social incompatibility, and inadequate response to intellectual, emotional, social, and physical demands without being grossly physically or mentally deficient upon examination. (Wolman, 1989, p. 250)

As used here, this term applies to those individuals who constantly measure themselves *upwards* against others (primarily among their peers who are more successful), and so come up failing or below them in all areas. Regardless of how well they do, they "should have done better." *Perfectionism* is part of their syndrome, and they never reach it. They are passive, compliant and willing to pay any price for acceptance and love (even though they realize it is not real!). They are constantly out to please others and attempt to *buy* their friendships, beginning as pre-school children and continuing into adulthood. Regardless of the methods employed, they never feel equal to others.

The main characteristic of this group of individuals is their compulsive need to measure and compare themselves to everyone else and come up failing. This need is so consistent and so all-pervasive that they will go to any lengths to assure their coming up short. Their negative self-image and defunct self-esteem have been present since early childhood, and are so ingrained that it is often next to impossible to change either.

As children, for example, these individuals may be able to name all the pupils in their class who scored higher than they did on a test, but are unconcerned about those who scored lower. They only measure upwards. If, by some happenstance, they score a 98% on a test, it should have been 100%; if they score 100%, the test was too easy! They never give themselves positive feedback or praise.

This compulsive need to compare and fail applies to all areas of their lives. They practice this degrading behavior in school, sports, and employment; in friendships and other relationships. The overall effect is a pervasive unhappy and depressed state. This eventually leads to social avoidance in all areas as a *safety* measure. They also start using the rationalization that "if I don't try, I can't fail."

BILLY: DEFECTIVE SELF-IMAGE INVITING MOLESTATION

An example, at this point, may be helpful:

☐ BILLY *comes home from school with his report card, containing seven A's and one C. With a great deal of anxiety, Billy hands the report card to his father who immediately responds: "What's that C doing there?" just as Billy knew he would and had done many times before. Billy does not respond but, with guilt and a deep sense of failure, goes to his room with one more confirmation that no matter what he does, he'll never be able to satisfy his father. Billy's father has taught him to see only the negative and to ignore the positive. The seven A's don't count, only the one C is important. Without any conscious standard of measurement or effort, this ruler is now firmly established and will remain there some 20 years later and be applied to everything he does, as we will see.*

The unfortunate, all-encompassing effect is that Billy may now see himself as below his peers in everything he does. Should he now get a 90% on a test and that turns out to be the highest grade in the class, his rationalization will be that he still should have gotten a 100%. Should he achieve the 100%, his rationalization will be that the test was too easy. While enjoying compliments at the moment they are given, he never internalizes them and remains, for all intents and purposes, incapable of seeing himself in a positive manner.

Billy also concludes that somehow, all of this *must be his fault*, since other fathers of his friends and classmates do not treat their sons in the same negative way. Eventually adopting his father's ruler, Billy becomes his own worst enemy. No matter how hard he tries, he never gives himself credit or praise, but through a distorted process that I call "subjective judgment" (further discussed in Chapter 5) he admires, respects, and praises the accomplishments of his friends and peers on a regular basis.

In my experience, *sex offenders handle criticism and insults far better than compliments or praise*, although the need for acceptance and approval simply gets stronger and stronger. This need also makes this type of child much more vulnerable to being victimized and used by both peers and adults. For this reason, they can easily become victims of sexual abuse early in their lives.

Continuing with this example:

Billy, as we have seen, cannot please his father, feels rejected and unloved and desperately needs a father's care and concern. His mother, also a very inadequate and frightened woman, cannot help Billy with his father's negative attitude. In an attempt to compensate for Billy's lost father's love, she enrolls Billy in the Big Brother program at the church she attends. She confides Billy's problems with his father to the intake-interviewer, and asks him for help. He readily agrees.

Billy reluctantly awaits his first contact with his new Big Brother, TOM, *predicting failure and ultimate rejection from this man, just as he received from his father. From the first week, Tom, to Billy, was a dream come true. Each week they went to movies, parks, on trips or for long walks. Tom took a personal and positive interest in Billy and was always touching him in one way or another. He put his arms around his shoulders, gave him hugs at their meeting and leaving, tousled his hair, etc. Billy had never received so much attention.*

After about a month, Tom suggested they take a weekend camping trip. Billy was thrilled, and his mother happily and readily gave her permission. On Friday afternoon, Billy and his new father substitute left for a state park.

During the trip, Tom rubbed Billy's leg and constantly found reasons for touching Billy. After setting up a tent in a secluded area of the park near the lake, Tom suggested a swim in their birthday suits and Billy agreed. At this point,

Billy would do anything to please Tom. In the waters of the lake, Tom again found reasons for touching and tickling, and explored Billy's body.

When they finished with the swim, Tom suggested they sunbathe to dry off and take a nap. Happy and tired, Billy fell asleep quite quickly and later awoke to Tom fellating him. Surprised, frightened and confused, Billy asked what Tom was doing, and his reply was: "Showing you how much I love you!" The sex act itself felt good and Billy simply laid back, eventually having his first orgasm. Tom asked nothing in return and the rest of the trip was fun and games.

However, from that trip on, each time Tom took Billy anywhere, they ended up at his apartment and, if it was a Friday, Billy slept over. The "love games," as the sexual molestations became known, not only continued but increased. Tom now wanted proof of Billy's love through reciprocal sex. The relationship continued for three years until Tom suddenly moved out of town. (Another boy had been molested and the Big Brother leadership asked Tom to resign or be reported to the police. In panic, Tom left town that weekend, without contacting Billy. The Big Brother leadership, embarrassed and fearing a potential law suit, never contacted Billy or his mother.) The results were devastating both then and some 12 years later when Billy, in the same manner, molested another young boy much like himself. Billy is now serving time for this offense.

THE EFFECT OF ADOLESCENT SEXUAL CRISIS

The sex offender personality typically behaves differently from the normal childhood personality. While both groups may experience similar behaviors due to their inadequate personalities, those who eventually become sex offenders also appear to experience some form of sexual trauma, active or passive, conscious or repressed, that, if unresolved, too often leads to sexual dysfunction and/or deviation in later life. As a result of lengthy experience with these individuals and with victims of sexual abuse who did not become sex offenders, we have derived some notions of how the two groups develop on different paths.

A schematic representation of this trait clearly shows how the early development of a negative, never-to-be-satisfied mental ruler separates the sex offender from the normal and natural progression of other children who experience this type of inadequate personality phase. The normals somehow adjust, get help or are helped through this state and tend to blossom at adolescence; the sex offender does not.

● A REPRESENTATION OF THE RELATIONSHIP BETWEEN CHILDHOOD PERSONALITY, SEXUAL CRISIS IN ADOLESCENCE, AND NORMAL OR PATHOLOGICAL SEXUAL ADJUSTMENT IN ADULTHOOD

☐ **The Basic Formula**

INADEQUATE PERSONALITY IN CHILDHOOD
+ SEXUAL TRAUMA IN CHILDHOOD OR ADOLESCENCE
[Conscious or repressed, Active or passive]
+ CRISIS, USUALLY AT PUBERTY
= ADULT OUTCOMES

ADULT OUTCOMES

☐ **DENY-ERS,** *WHO CONTROL AND OVERCOMPENSATE*
♦ *NON-SEXUALLY:*
→ NON-CRIMINALLY, THROUGH SPORTS, POWER, MONEY
→ CRIMINALLY, AS WIFE-BEATERS, MUGGERS, ASSAULTIVE PERSONALITIES
♦ *SEXUALLY*
→ NON-CRIMINALLY, AS PLAYBOYS, LADY'S MEN, MACHO PERSONALITIES
→ CRIMINALLY, THROUGH SEXUALLY ASSAULTIVE BEHAVIOR AGAINST CHILDREN OR ADULTS

☐ **ADJUST-ERS,** *WHO GET HELP THROUGH COUNSELING OR THERAPY OR POSITIVE LIFE EXPERIENCES AND THUS MATURE*

☐ **ACCEPT-ERS**
♦ *NON-SEXUALLY:*
→ NON-CRIMINALLY, BY BECOMING MAMA'S BOYS, HAPPY HEN-PECKED HUSBANDS, OR GENERALLY PASSIVE PERSONS [E.G., THE LAST CLERK IN THE OFFICE SYNDROME]
→ CRIMINALLY, THROUGH EMBEZZLING, ARSON, FRAUD, AND OTHER NON-CONTACT OFFENSES
♦ *SEXUALLY:*
→ NON-CRIMINALLY, AS PASSIVE HOMOSEXUALS, PERENNIAL BACHELORS, VOLUNTARY CELIBATES
→ CRIMINALLY, AS SEDUCTIVE PEDOPHILES OR HEBOPHILES, FLASHERS WHO CONTROL IN THIS MANNER

For both groups of children, a *crisis* occurs at adolescence, precipitated by the beginnings of self-evaluation, comparison to peers and a dramatic change in the source of their social and acceptance needs. While as children they wanted and needed to please adults for approval, security and acceptance, they now change to wanting to please peers and seek acceptance, security and approval from this group.

Identity, instead of being linked to the father-ideal figure (for boys), now shifts to admiration for the peer-model who is accepted, popular and assertive, as well as successful in the eyes of the newcomer.

The normal adolescent simply enters a new stage of life and smoothly adjusts with little visible trauma (except possibly for his parents). He joins his peer group and quickly establishes a new identity, different from childhood, and continues to grow and mature as he encounters new and challenging experiences, sexual awakening and plans for the future.

MODES OF PATHOLOGICAL ADJUSTMENT IN ADULTHOOD

For the potential sex offender, the already established negative ruler determines the course he will take. He responds to the adolescent crisis in a totally different manner and comes to a crossroad where he can go in only one of two directions and become either:

- The *deny-er*, by definition, cannot face the perceived inadequacy. Through reaction-formation and denial he overcompensates for the inadequacy either:

[1] *Legally* through excelling in sports, power, wealth, "macho" behaviors and persistent proofs of his physical and sexual prowess. There are never enough of these successes and each one triggers an even stronger need for more and more proof until the behaviors become compulsive; *or*

[2] *Illegally* through rape, wife-abuse, breaking and entering, daring and risky robberies, etc., again to prove his masculinity and, now, his superiority over his peers. However, as stated above, the overcompensation never works and never ends, increasing in intensity, violence, and daring.

- An example of the deny-er (legally) might easily be the playboy who has to have a different conquest each night; consistently needs a high-rating of his sexual performance; brags continuously to fellow workers of his latest sexual success, and who, simultaneously, is overly competitive in the workplace, throwing ethics out the window in order to advance and to win out over everyone, including his supervisor. He also has to act at being happy since he never really is.

- An example of the deny-er (illegally) is the rapist who is never satisfied with his sexual performance or a willing and cooperative partner but must take what he wants and cause pain while doing it. In therapy, the rapist will frequently allude to the partial motivation that he wanted someone else to feel the pain he felt all of his life.

- Another pertinent example would be the incestuous father who must rule the lives of his family as a dictator to prove his control, power and worth. Regardless of how the family tries to please this individual, they cannot succeed and he steadily graduates from physical and financial control to sexual control over his wife and his children.

- The *accept-er* who accepts his situation and comes to the conclusion quite early in life that he will never change, and never meet his or anyone else's expectations. As a result, he does nothing to alleviate his state. He then either:

[1] *Legally* (sexually) becomes the passive homosexual who does anything to please his partner (usually a dominant figure similar to his father) and is never secure in his relationship. He usually destroys the relationship with his insecurity, jealousy and suspicions of betrayal, literally pushing his partner away, in order to confirm the predicted rejection. Non-sexually, he becomes the happily henpecked husband or remains the momma's boy, quits easily at everything he attempts (one strike and he quits the team; one bad grade or recitation in school and he quits the class), or becomes the clerk in the fiftieth desk of an office where the fiftieth desk is the lowest. His goal there is to work for 20 years, possibly getting to the forty-ninth desk and retiring with his gold watch. These individuals will be relatively happy with their lot, since it poses no risk of failure that any change, promotion or advancement would. Were his supervisor, for example, to pick him out for training for a higher level position, he would perceive it akin to being asked to jump off the World Trade Center and fly. He would also probably quit and run away since *escape* is his main protective defense and coping mechanism — *or*

[2] *Illegally* (sexually) he becomes the child molester (either pedophile or hebophile, depending on the degree of inadequacy or the

age bracket of his own sexual molestation) or the exhibitionist. Non-sexually he becomes the arsonist, embezzler, or the bookie or he may choose many other non-contact forms of criminal behavior.

Even in the case of the child molester, his need is to please the child, not himself, and quite often he performs on the child not expecting or asking for reciprocal pleasure.

HOWIE: THE ULTIMATE INADEQUATE PERSONALITY

An example of this type of individual is HOWIE, one of the most difficult cases that I have ever encountered.

☐ *Howie was a momma's boy who lived in a totally matriarchal household with a passive, almost non-existent older father. All of his life, his need was to please mother. At college-age, Howie was incapable of making a decision, never had a true friend nor was ever involved in an equal relationship.*

Howie chose teaching as a career and grammar school as the level he would teach. He felt safe in this environment and did not see the young children as a threat. From the beginning of his teaching career, he felt strangely attracted to young boys. His primary attractions were all to what he termed Adonises who were also the most popular boys in the class and the school.

Howie, being a loner most of his life, chose photography as a substitute social life and slowly but surely talked several of the young boys into posing nude for him on field trips and camping weekends (which he supervised for the nature club). He never touched any of the boys, although he did get erections seeing them naked. Only after years of therapy could he even admit to himself that there was a sexual attraction or component to his behavior. Howie also never masturbated until he was 31 years old, when he saw one boy do it in the woods and then imitated the behavior. Were it not for a nosy relative who went into his darkroom and rifled through his photos, discovering the pictures of the nude boys, Howie would never have been caught. It is doubtful that he would have progressed to actual physical contact or overt sexual behavior since his fears of both physical contact and sex were so paralyzing and since he was so content with what he had — the photos.

Howie's long-term, difficult treatment will be discussed in the section on treatment techniques.

It must be noted here that the *pervasive and omnipresent inade-quacy* may not always easily be seen, especially in the deny-ers. Their social and work images are carefully rehearsed and orchestrated to prevent their true nature (their inadequate personality) from being seen or discovered. They work very hard to create the image of normalcy, aptitude and expertise in their vocation. This applies especially to the professional groups (teachers, ministers of all denominations, scoutmasters, big brothers, policemen, doctors, lawyers, psychiatrists/psychologists, etc.).

One *key* to their diagnosis and detection, if one looks for it, is that while they always seem to know a great deal about their colleagues and fellow workers, no one interviewed knows anything really personal about their private lives outside the workplace. They rarely, if ever, have a real friendship or relationship on an intimate level.

FRANK: OVER-COMPENSATION FOR SEXUAL VICTIMIZATION

An example of two such offenders might help to clarify this phenomenon:

☐ FRANK *was a very popular child, good athlete and honor student, both in grammar school and in high school. His parents had no complaints about his behavior at home and, in every way, Frank was considered a normal boy. Frank successfully hid both his feelings of inadequacy and need to excel to make up for these feelings, as well as his anger and hatred for all women.*

Early in Frank's life (when he was around eight years old), he was sexually molested by a teenage female babysitter who undressed him and herself, had him lick her vagina (which was not too clean) and then laughed and ridiculed him about his then small penis. Frank could not perform to her satisfaction and could not please her, although he desperately wanted to. She concluded the molestation with the traumatizing statement: "Kid, you'll never be a real man and you'll never be able to please a woman!"

Frank never forgot the experience or the babysitter's words, but was too frightened and embarrassed to tell anyone about it. Concurrently, he had problems with his two older sisters, who picked on him and resented the fact that they had to babysit for him when their parents went out. The two sisters physically abused him: pinching him, tickling him until he cried, spanking him, naked, with a hairbrush and also laughing at his small penis, which they went out of their way to focus on and ridicule.

When he entered adolescence, Frank's attitude was "love them and leave them" and his intercourse with any woman was brutal and aimed to cause pain. Threats were used to keep all of his secrets. In the sports locker rooms he always had an excuse not to shower with the other players, but still was sure to check them out and compare himself, especially genitally. Naturally, he always came out lacking.

In his first and all subsequent employments, Frank was an excellent and diligent worker, always exceeding what was asked of him and always competing with the other workers. Although he was socially friendly on the surface, no one really knew much about Frank's private life, but that was okay with his friends.

Frank was known as a lady's man and was always seen with a different date. He had grown into a good-looking, muscular hunk on the outside but inside he was still a small, weak and frightened little boy. After a particularly important date on which he experienced impotence and was ridiculed for it, all of the "old tapes" began to play. After brooding for hours, he went out in the middle of the night and committed his first brutal rape. The victim was a young college woman, hitchhiking home from studying with a friend. She was subsequently hospitalized for her injuries and required plastic surgery on her face. She never again returned to college and is still in psychotherapy.

Frank's rapes continued for more than three years before he was caught. During that time, he associated with many policemen and discussed the rapes with them and also with his friends at work. His attitude was always one of horror and disgust toward the rapist and he adamantly insisted that the animal should be castrated or killed when caught. Never was Frank suspected and when he was finally apprehended and identified by one victim, no one, including his policemen friends, believed the story. The whole community came to his defense. Only after he finally confessed out of guilt and to experience some relief, did his true personality become known, even to his own family.

Howie (whom we have already met) was a certified grammar school teacher. He was well liked by the students and also by the teachers who elected him their union representative. While he attended all school social functions and even dated one of the teachers (a frightening and unpleasant experience as he was later to relate), he had no real, intimate friends and, as with Frank, no one really knew anything about his personal life except that he was dedicated to teaching and to his students. He was labeled by one of his administrators as: "Almost too good to be true" and this certainly proved to be the case. At hearing of his arrest, all who knew him were shocked. His parents (especially his mother), to this day, refuse to believe the extent of his pathology or the number of children he was involved with (more than 100 over four years). Howie chose the perfect place to hide his truly inadequate personality, a grammar school. There was no competition for him to be concerned with and he certainly physically could handle sixth graders.

Both Howie and Frank are typical sex offenders and their cases are in no way unique. Due to the ability of the sex offender to hide and compensate for his pathology, sex offenders are invisible threats and not easily screened out of the situations that both feed and satisfy their illness! In subsequent chapters, we will meet many other cases of this kind.

3

The Never-Satisfied Parent:
Negative Self-Image and
Selective Perception

Add to the already basic inadequate personality a never-satisfied parent and the overall effect can be and usually is devastating. In every aspect of the developing sex offender personality, the results are the same: negative. Whether in school performance, sports, social events, family behavior or physical development (size, strength, appearance, body image) our subject perceives himself to be at the bottom of the totem pole and erroneously concludes that he will never measure up.

Then, through an identification with the never-to-be-satisfied parent, the sex offender becomes his own worst enemy. From childhood on, no matter what he does, it is never good enough to satisfy either his perfectionistic parent(s) or his own perfectionistic self.

KEVIN: PROGRESSION FROM EXHIBITION TO VIOLENT RAPE

☐ KEVIN *is a very bright and creative adult (WAIS Full Scale I.Q. = 157) who is a compulsive rapist. After some time in his first treatment experience (he is presently a parole violator from the state of Massachusetts and again is incarcerated), Kevin unexpectedly joined the arts and crafts program at the institution where he was being treated. He displayed a truly remarkable talent in both painting and sculpture. His works were originals (many others in the program copied from books, great artists, etc.) and showed a warmth and sensitivity not seen in his daily behavior or in any of his therapy modalities. Both staff and patients admired his works and often came to him for advice, suggestions and help when their projects were not going well. He gladly helped and seemed to enjoy doing so.*

One day, during a therapy session, Kevin asked his therapist to keep one of his works in his office and the therapist agreed. The therapist also commented enthusiastically on the rich quality, the creative flair, and the originality of the painting. Kevin immediately went on a tirade about the flaws in the picture: proportional problems, poor color choices, etc. It was obvious that he was extremely uncomfortable with the praise he had received and needed to negate it as quickly as possible. While he could identify his own reaction as coming from what he expected from his father as a child, this insight did not alter his critical opinion of the painting. He withdrew his request to hang the picture in the therapist's office and left with the painting. It was never seen again.

This was typical behavior for Kevin, as it is for the majority of sex offenders. They receive some instant gratification from praise and support then a form of panic sets in and their perfectionism takes over. It is almost as if they fear any positive comment, while underneath they yearn for it.

PERFECTIONISM AND THE FEAR OF FAILURE SYNDROME

Perfectionism, then, becomes a paramount therapeutic concern and barrier to be surmounted. The patient's perfectionism needs to be replaced with a more realistic appraisal of their lives and ultimately of themselves.

A *fear of failure syndrome* develops as a natural consequence of the perfectionism and becomes exaggerated to the point where fear of trying becomes phobically entrenched. Cognitions attached to this syndrome include:

- "If I try, I'll fail and then I'll feel even worse about myself than I do now, so it's better not even to try," or
- "I'll take a risk but as soon as I get scared or start to fail, I'll quit and run for the safety of not ever trying again."

Thus, if such a patient is talked into going back to school (as an adult), he may quit at the first sign of an unacceptable teacher (parent substitute) response, and never return. Similarly, if he joins a softball team and, when up to bat, hears *"Strike one!"*, he throws down the bat, turns in his uniform and quits the team.

Although the above two examples may seem exaggerated, I have seen them both occur hundreds of times in sex offenders. Whether encouraged to become involved in school, a sports program, art programs, new groups, volunteer activities, approaching an authority figure, or any other activity that is perceived as a risk, the sex offender will avoid these activities at all costs.

Fear of failure, more than any other factor makes motivating the sex offender very difficult, especially when it involves taking risks by exposing himself in group. It can take as long as seven to ten years of passive silence and high levels of resistance before any really meaningful therapy takes place. Thus the essential need for patience on the part of therapists choosing to work with this population.

The more inadequate and the more pathological the offender is, the more he resists and the more time that will be needed to see even the most simple changes and/or gains. For some offenders, fear of failure is so all-encompassing and so paralyzing that they never participate in therapy to a meaningful degree, nor do they ever expose what is really going on in their thoughts, fantasies, etc. In addition, they never discuss the childhood traumas or experiences that led to their deviation. Effective therapy under these circumstances does not exist. The real danger here is that *confinement increases their illness, whether their pervasive inadequacy or their suppressed rage, and they eventually return to society more dangerous than when they were first confined.*

There appears also to be a direct correlation between the degree of resistance and the degree of abuse they incurred as children or adolescents.

During his first sentence to the treatment program, Kevin denied any real pathology or problems and projected all blame onto his parents, especially his demanding and unsatisfied father. In treatment, while being willing to participate and to help others, he was unwilling to expose his own personal and deep-seated problems. At the end of three years, he was released, now more dangerous than when he arrived as a flasher. Exposure to therapy had brought many old memories and traumas to consciousness, and his already deep sense of inadequacy increased.

Shortly following release he began flashing again but now with fantasies of rape, as opposed to his former fantasies of seduction. Within the first several months of his return to the community he met a woman (with whom he was not compatible), and after a brief courtship married her against the advice of his family and his outpatient therapist. Within a year of the marriage, Kevin began raping and accumulated over 60 victims before he was eventually discovered.

TODD: A VICTIM OF INCEST WHO BECOMES A SERIAL RAPIST

A different example will help to clarify the concept:

☐ TODD *spent most of his adolescence and young adult years in trouble with the law and either on probation or in an institution of one type or another. When I first met him, he was sentenced to 30 years for rape. Todd was likable, a good inmate and popular with both the staff and his peers. He had a great deal of talent in the electronics area and was assigned to work in the maintenance department of the video studio complex.*

In therapy he was passive and rarely participated in group, either for himself or others. In individual therapy, he was a bit more involved, but participated only in answer to direct questions. After more than a year, he began to open up more and one day related that he had been sexually molested at age 12 by an older brother. Their sexual behavior began with Todd being talked into masturbating his brother (with no reciprocation). In return the brother allowed Todd to drive his car, join him on camping or hunting trips, and to hang-out with the brother's older friends. Todd felt accepted and was willing to pay for this acceptance and involvement.

Not too long after their sexual involvement began, Todd's brother changed the format of the sexual behavior, and painfully sodomized Todd. Both during and after the sodomy, his brother compared Todd favorably to the girls he had. This increased the degree of trauma for Todd but once hooked on the benefits of submitting, he could not refuse and was at the mercy of his brother's frustrated sex life. Almost concurrently, Todd's school grades and behavior deteriorated. He became quiet and withdrawn, socially isolated from his former age-mates and spent all of his time either with his older brother or doing favors and chores for him.

The only reason Todd brought this trauma up in individual therapy was that he was bleeding rectally from inserting objects into his anus for pleasure. He was at a point where he could not masturbate to orgasm without something inserted up his rectum. Shame, disgust and fear also motivated him to bring the subject up. I referred him to the hospital for treatment, and although the physician warned him of the dangers of continuing this practice, Todd ignored the warning saying that he could not stop.

TREATMENT CONSIDERATIONS

For the particular problem of failure-phobia that the sex offender invariably brings into therapy (as do many survivors of
sexual abuse), one early and very important treatment goal should
be to encourage risk-taking activities and behaviors that are likely
to result in success.

To begin this process, *goals are set that ensure success with little or
no chance of failure.* Building on some base of an already familiar
behavior, improvement goals are set extremely low to prevent
failure. Two examples will clarify:

- Let us say that one of the offenders in a therapist's caseload is interested
  in improving his physical condition and wants to do some running of
  laps on the gymnasium's track. He tells you that yesterday he ran two
  laps of the track and will run again today. The natural tendency would
  be to either repeat the goal of two laps or to increase the goal to at least
  three laps. With this type of individual, both of these goals are dangerous and could produce a failure that surely would result in his ending
  this activity. Therefore, he is taught to set his next goal at one lap. Thus,
  if he runs two laps again, he has exceeded his goal and that becomes a
  bonus that he must accept as both positive and a success. The same for
  three or even four laps.

- If the goal for the offender is to reduce his isolation and fear of talking
  to others on his housing wing or place of employment in the community, the initial goal would be to come out of his room or workspace at
  least one time during the morning, afternoon and evening and say
  "Hi!" to one other person. If he speaks to two or more individuals or
  becomes involved in a lengthy conversation, this is a bonus that must
  be seen as positive and a success.

This *minimal goal-setting below the client's true ability* technique
works with all offenders who are willing to try it, whether in an
institution or in the community. The technique applies to all
phases of the offender's life. As self- confidence increases, the
therapist may then suggest attempts at behaviors that are more
related to the offender's specific problems or fears. However, here
again, each new behavior demands the same *setting himself up to
succeed* technique.

Caveat: In using this technique it is extremely important to begin
these new behaviors with choices that the offender has some

knowledge of and some former experience with. Beginning new and unfamiliar behaviors *before self- confidence is firmly established* can confirm his old perception of being a failure and worthless and therefore must be avoided.

As with all techniques, there will be times when even this minimal goal setting system fails. These situations afford the therapist the opportunity to alter an old perception of failure: Replace "Failure is painful, embarrassing, depressing and to be avoided at all costs" with: "Failure is positive!" When the client looks at you as if you had lost your senses, you simply ask him to explain your statement. Eventually, they all come to realize that the reason failure is positive is twofold: you can learn from your mistakes, but more importantly: in order to fail, you had to try or you had to take a risk and that is always a positive. Sex offenders are able to identify with this second factor quite easily since trying has been one of their greatest deficits.

From *performance behaviors,* the next progression in the process is to *interpersonal behaviors* where the offender perceives the greatest risk-taking to exist. Depending on the case and the individual, these might include:

- Making a new friend or associate.
- Beginning to share more personal information about himself with one person.
- Taking the floor more frequently in group.
- Beginning to share frightening or embarrassing secrets with the therapist and eventually the group.
- Sharing feelings with just one person.
- Saying "No," possibly for the first time in their lives to someone they fear loosing as a friend or parent- substitute (such as the therapist).
- Asking for advice and then following their own decision anyway. This is a very important step in their progress.
- Admitting the offense with full responsibility rather than rationalizing, projecting or denying.
- Increasing socialization behaviors and increasing their circle of friends and associates.

- Where appropriate, confronting individuals in their lives who have negatively affected them, hurt them or possibly abused them either physically or sexually.

Personal growth and self-confidence result, slowly but definitely as these exercises continue and become more daring. The reward is the formation of a new and stronger ego (self) that is decidedly necessary if the offender is to succeed.

At this level of progress, a major caveat is necessary: The overall and ultimate goal of these treatment techniques is the formation of a new and functional personality structure. Since the choice of what will embody this new personality is the offender's decision, the therapist must be cautious of how this choice is made.

NEW IMAGE DANGERS

Becoming What Others Want

For most of their lives, especially as children, sex offenders were total conformists to others' wishes in order to gain the acceptance and love they so desperately craved. This survival behavior pattern will not be extinguished overnight. In fact, residual elements of this behavior will unconsciously recur on a regular basis and the offender must be consistently made aware of each occurrence.

Not only does this danger apply to his new image but it also is extremely important in any new career choice(s). Many (if not the majority of) offenders have chosen to follow the occupation or trade of their fathers, brothers, uncles, grandfathers or some other significant influence in their lives. Often the result is disastrous with the offender either failing in this chosen field or hating it and living unhappily. The same danger applies to choosing a new personality. A statements such as: "My father always wanted me to be tough and strong and assertive" is indicative of this syndrome.

Imitating an Idol

In a similar manner, when there is no one in the family that the offender wants to imitate, the next choice they tend to make is to become like someone they idolize, respect, admire. It could be the therapist, a close friend they have known for years, someone they met in their group, or simply someone who symbolizes all that they have always wanted to be and could not be. Examples of this syndrome might include statements such as: "I'd like to be like my father or my brother," or "If only I could be as tough and assertive as my uncle John" are indicative of this syndrome.

Becoming the Opposite of "Their Old Selves"

This is probably the second worst choice that the offender could make. Being someone whose thinking is all black and white (extremes) and who has problems with gray areas (moderate) is one of the offender's major problems. If this occurs, the therapist's function is to help the offender find positive facets of his personality that work well for him and that he should retain in his new personality development. In my experience, I have never met an offender who was all bad and who did not possess many positive traits, talents, skills, values and behaviors.

For example, the majority of the offenders I have worked with have been excellently skilled either in some professional area such as teaching, the ministry, or even counseling or in some business or technical field such as electronics, computer programming or repair, construction even finance. (Very few sex offenders that I have encountered were day workers or nomadic types.)

There is always a way to utilize these valuable skills in their new lives. Some (such as teachers, ministers and priests) will be unable to return to their former profession or employment. However, there is no reason that a former grammar school teacher could not become a vocational-technical teacher with adults or even teach in a junior college, college or business school.

Many that I have treated have done just that and were successful at it. Priests and ministers, while they may not be allowed to return to active parish level work where they have contact with children, adolescents or young adults, can certainly teach in seminaries or theological colleges. These possibilities must be carefully pointed out to the offender with the caveat that the choice must remain his.

Staying the Same

Fear of taking risks is paramount in the offender group. They have consistently failed so often throughout their lives that they anticipate failure at every new venture. The result is that it is easier to stay the same because it's safe and comfortable. Moving the offender from this position is probably the greatest challenge that the therapist will meet. The old embedded value *"once a— always a— !"* returns over and over again, and the resistance to replacing this value with a more realistic one is tremendous.

Small, new, risk-taking behaviors, with minimal danger and little or no consequence for failure, become primary homework assignments that *must* be part of the offender's treatment. These assignments should begin almost from the first session. They should be consistently given at the end of each session and then evaluated at the beginning of the next session. If the outcome was positive, realistic praise and reinforcement should be given; if the offender failed, then an analysis of *why* he failed becomes the focus of the first part of the therapy session. Either way the assignments must continue until he is able to set goals of this type on his own.

"I Don't Deserve to Change"

When this barrier to a new personality is encountered, it indicates that guilt is still so overpowering that any attempts at making changes at this juncture are doomed to failure. Thus, the "new personality development phase" must be suspended and the total focus of treatment aimed at resolving the degree of guilt present, its origin, the values associated with it and the means to assuage it. Until the level of guilt is reduced to a level where the offender feels that he is deserving of positive feedback without becoming self-destructive, no further therapy goals can be set or activated.

"I Don't Believe Change is Possible for Me"

Here, the double standard of the sex offender is alive and well. While he is willing to admit that change for everyone else in the world is possible, he perceives it as impossible for himself. From my personal experience, I feel strongly that this barrier is closely tied in with the prior one of being undeserving. In fact, the two appear to be intimately linked. In most cases, resolving the degree and level of perceived guilt is sufficient to resolve this barrier and allow the new personality development to proceed.

Incidentally, these *new image dangers* are also found in the treatment of the survivors of sexual abuse and the procedures for resolving them are practically identical.

SELECTIVE PERCEPTION

A characteristic of the offender that accounts for many of the problems just discussed is *selective perception,* one of the most startling traits found in these individuals and traceable to his youth. This term refers to the ability to block out parts of reality that do not conform to the need to constantly measure upward and to compare unfavorably to the peer group.

An example may help to clarify this concept:

☐ *One late afternoon as I was about to leave a junior high school, where I was employed part time as a psychological consultant, the principal asked me to see just one more young man who had always been a polite, scholarly and very popular individual during his grammar school years, but who suddenly had become a habitual truant. Tired after a full day, I tried to postpone the case until my next scheduled appointment day. However, the principal insisted that I see* RONNY *today since, if he were truant one more time, he would be reported to the authorities and would possibly end up in a reformatory. I agreed.*

When Ronny entered my office, I observed a well-developed, handsome young man who had knocked on the door, called me "sir" when asking to enter and appeared to be a polite and mannerly individual. Tired and pressed for time, I went straight to the heart of the matter and stated: "Look, Ronny, I really don't have a great deal of time to listen to a long story. Just tell me what I can do to get you back into classes and we'll get along fine." He immediately said: "Get me out of gym classes."

After a moment I agreed and wrote him a note on my stationery, excusing him from gym classes until further notice. He immediately asked , "What's the trick, Doc?" I stated that there was no trick and that I understood how he felt since he must have the smallest penis in the class. He asked "How did you know that?" I did not respond and he continued: "And that's not all; guess what my nickname is? Bald eagle!" Noticing his closely cropped crewcut, I told him that I thought it looked fine, and he informed me that I was looking in the wrong place and pointed to his crotch. He then explained that he was the only boy in his gym class who was totally hairless, while all the others were not only larger in all ways but also had pubic hair.

At this point, I asked Ronny for a favor. I needed him to return to his gym class just one more time and in the shower to check out all of the other boys, in case there was another boy with a similar problem. While he assured me that there wasn't anyone else like him in the class, he agreed. The next day, Ronny came knocking on the door, yelling "Doc! Doc! you won't believe what happened!" He then related that he had done as I had asked and that there were five more "bald eagles" and that, even more startling, there were three boys with penises as small or even smaller than his. With a very serious face, I asked: "Ronny, why did you lie to me the last time we met?" With the most sincere facial and vocal expression I had seen or heard in quite a while (pay close attention to his answer) Ronny stated: "I swear, Doc, they weren't there the other times."

As one might guess, they had been there. However, by a mechanism I term selective perception, Ronny measured himself upwards only and perceptually blocked out the other similar or even smaller boys until specifically directed to take notice of them.

This same phenomenon occurs in all other areas of the sex offenders' lives, from home where they measure against siblings and parents, to society, school and all other situations where comparison or measurement occurs.

Selective perception is another of the factors that makes treating either the sex offender or the victim of sex offenses so difficult and meticulous a task. All through the therapy process, whenever the patient becomes self-judgmental, this factor must be looked for and eliminated before moving any further. His perception of himself is continually colored and distorted by this factor, and to move past even the smallest judgmental statement without checking it's validity can affect the remainder of the session and even alter the course of therapy. Selective perception must be dealt with as early as possible during therapy. Specific techniques will be discussed in later chapters.

4

Exaggerated Needs for Control

Control is a constant and dominant factor in the overwhelming preponderance of sex offenses, regardless of the type of act or the age of the victim. The ways in which the need to control may be expressed in antisocial sexual behavior are presented in a schematic format on the next page that offers a diagram of how such control needs may be expressed by degrees, from minimal control to total control.

CONTROL METHODS OF EXHIBITIONISTS AND VOYEURS

Even in noncontact sex offenses, such as exhibitionism, control exists. As soon as the offender gets the intended victim(s) to look at his exposed genitals, a smile appears on his face, the cognition "Gotcha!" or "Made you look!" occurs, and his satisfaction begins, even if he gets no further with his behavior. Should the victim smile and approach (if the fantasy was seductive), or scream, run or indicate fear (if the fantasy was assaultive), the pleasure is even greater.

In the case of voyeurism, the counterpart of exhibitionism, the control factor is found in the fantasy: if the offender is a *deny-er*, this will be a force and rape type fantasy; if he is an *accept-er*, there will be a successful seduction fantasy.

- **THREE AVENUES THROUGH WHICH SEXUAL DEVIATES EXPRESS THEIR NEEDS TO CONTROL ANOTHER PERSON**

  ☐ **Using Force And Violence To Express Anger And Hatred Towards The Victim Through:**
  - → SEXUAL HARASSMENT
  - → FLASHING AND/OR OBSCENE PHONE CALLS, WITH RAPE OR ASSAULT FANTASIES
  - → FORCED ACTS OF FELLATIO, CUNNILINGUS, ANAL SEX, UROPHILIA, INTERCOURSE

  ☐ **Using Violence And Terror By Denigrating The Victim Through:**
  - → SADISTIC INJURY TO BREASTS, SEXUAL ORGANS
  - → SEXUAL MURDER

  ☐ **Using Seduction To Satisfy Their Need For Acceptance As:**
  - → A SEDUCTIVE PEDOPHILE/HEBOPHILE, PASSIVE HOMOSEXUAL, FLASHER, PEEPING TOM, or OBSCENE PHONE CALLER WITH SEDUCTION FANTASIES

CONTROL METHODS OF PEDOPHILES AND HEBOPHILES

The pedophile or hebophile exerts control over victims in many ways, not only when they succeed in a sexual sense but also in other aspects of the victims lives, making the victim dependent on the offender for love, affection, support, etc. Once the victim is hooked, the offender can then become more bold and more overtly sexual in his behavior toward him/her.

DON: A LONG-TIME PEDOPHILE

When the child/adolescent becomes older and more independent and the offender feels his control is slipping, the victim is dropped and replaced by another, more inadequate and dependent one and the cycle begins again. This "seducing/dropping" phenomenon accounts for the very large number of victims this particular group eventually accumulates. An example may clarify this concept:

☐ DON *is the sixth grade teacher in an elementary school, where the sixth grade is the last and highest grade. From there, the children go on to a junior high school across town. During the first week of each semester, Don, a longtime pedophile, begins the selection process of his victims for that school year. In his mind, he is looking for a specific type of boy: one who is cute and good-looking, friendly and somewhat assertive, has a minimal closeness to his father, is popular with the other students and, most importantly, will probably need extra help during the school year. He finds five or six each school year.*

Slowly, over the next several months (no fewer than three) Don develops a special relationship with each of the boys, independently of the others. He assigns them special jobs in the classroom, finds excuses for them to stay after school and makes sure that they know he is their friend and wants to help them. When he feels comfortable enough with any of them, he offers them tutoring at his apartment. One of the most shocking elements of these molestations is the ease with which Don and others like him are able to get the parents' permission for this type of activity, simply because he is a teacher — even though the parents have never met him.

The first session at the apartment is legitimate and very positively and supportively oriented. Don suggests that several more sessions would be beneficial and the boys each agreed. Don makes sure that the second or third session lasts until dinner time and then calls the parents, telling them how great things are progressing and suggesting that he be allowed to take the boy to McDonald's for supper. He says that it would also be beneficial if they continued tutoring after dinner since things were going so well. If the parents sound pleased, he then suggests that the boy be allowed to sleep over and that he will bring him to school. Surprisingly, he never had a parent refuse!

After another half-hour or so of tutoring, Don suggests they need some fun and suggest card-playing, which he eventually leads to strip poker. He makes sure he loses the first game to test the boy's reaction to nudity and, if the boy reacts with interest, laughing, etc., he makes sure the boy loses the next game. Next in the well-planned scenario is Polaroid picture-taking, followed by tickling when both he and the boy are nude, and mild groping. If all goes well, that ends this night's adventure for Don.

Over the next few tutoring sessions, Don begins asking questions about sex and masturbation and begins to teach a sex education course, sometimes bringing his five or six chosen boys together for the first time. Don extols the joys and need for masturbation to become a normal, healthy man and from here on the progression is predictable: self- masturbation to mutual masturbation to contests of speed, first ejaculator, etc. All during this process the Polaroids continue and now become both security and a pressure tool to advance the deviant behavior even further to fellatio, etc.

Don's behavior went on for several years, lasting only with each group of boys for one school year. Don felt that this practice would provide safety for him since his was the last grade in his school and the following year the boys were transferred to a junior high school across town. Each year he seduced a new group of boys (usually about five or six) and this behavior continued for four years before he was exposed.

One day, one of his boys acted up in class and became openly defiant. Don kept him after school and the parents then threatened to severely punish the boy for his behavior that embarrassed and shamed them. In anger and in defense, the boy related what Don had done to him and connected it to the school punishment. Subsequently Don was arrested and confessed to the true number involved: a minimum of 40 victims over a period of ten years.

The school authorities were shocked as were his fellow teachers. All insisted that there "wasn't the slightest clue or hint of Don's secret life or deviant tendencies." Part of this was due to the fact that for several years of his teaching career, Don had been married and appeared to be the typical middle-class person in his neighborhood and at all school social functions, which he usually chaired. Don's wife reported normal sexual behavior and a good marital relationship for the first year or so, but then his work and devotion to the school and the kids overshadowed their lives. What she did not know was that even during their sex, Don was fantasizing being with one of his boys.

THE DECEPTION WAS ALMOST PERFECT

Don's background is quite interesting: Don's first sexual knowledge occurred at age 12 with an older female cousin after they had been swimming. She undressed herself and Don, had him lay on top of her, put his penis in her and that was it. When Don was 13, a male cousin, age 14, returned from camping and told Don that in his cabin they had had contests to see who had the most pubic hair, and that he always won. He asked to see Don's and when Don dropped his shorts, they first compared and then "he played with mine and I played with his and I liked it!" Their sex play continued and progressed to mutual masturbation, then oral sex, then intercrural intercourse. Don liked it all because: "it felt good!" Don claimed that "he showed me the attention and acceptance that I never had before from anyone!" Then Don and his family moved to a new neighborhood: "The people next door had an older boy and my cousin and I got involved with him. They had a clubhouse and I asked him if he had ever done anything sexual and from there we progressed to what I had done with my cousin plus mutual sodomy." This went on for a couple of years and the imprint (see Chapter 14) occurred.

During this period, Don engaged in some petting with girls but nothing else since he "wasn't interested." He feared if he tried to go any further with a girl, she would know from his behavior (and probable failure) that he was a homosexual. In college, Don had intercourse with a woman for the first time: "It was okay but no where near as enjoyable as my homosexual experiences. I felt I had to perform with girls, but with boys I never did."

Don's masturbation continued during this time but only with homosexual fantasies. They always involved either his cousin or the boy next door or both. In Vietnam, Don went to the bath houses and paid for oral sex from the prostitutes but never went any further. He wanted to have sex with many of his army friends and mates but was too afraid of exposure and rejection.

Don married at age 30, more out of societal pressure than desire or love. Sex was "okay" but again "never as good as the homosexual experiences."

His first molestation of a youngster occurred at the end of his first year of teaching, before he was married. At first he limited himself to fondling but when the boy said he liked it and that he had been fellating other boys in the class (according to Don); Don felt this was the green light and went further. Their sexual relationship lasted from May to October and then stopped when the boy told other kids in the class and told Don that he didn't want to do it anymore (probably due to the reaction of his peers).

Don's marriage lasted one and a half years and ended in divorce. Six months after the divorce he went to kids again and this continued with his students for four years until he was arrested. Don had, by then, molested over 40 young boy students in his charge.

Don's inadequacy can be traced all the way back to childhood. He never felt equal to or comfortable with peers and schoolmates until the sexual incidents. This was the only place he felt comfortable and accepted.

Later in life, whenever he was under pressure or felt that he had failed (usually following a personal rejection) he reverted to his former inadequate self and immediately became obsessed with the sexual fantasies from the past and the need to reenact those pleasurable behaviors. He accomplished this by regressing to the age at which these experiences occurred and then looking for a playmate to have sex with.

Don vividly recalled taking some boys to Great Adventure Amusement Park and riding all the rides with them, "feeling like I was 11 years old again. All fun, no responsibilities, someone paying the way and free!"

This delusional regression to the child's age when everything was fun and games is quite typical of both the pedophile and the hebophile.

CONTROL METHODS IN SEXUALLY ASSAULTIVE PERSONS

Where rape behavior or other forms of sexual assault are concerned the control factor is obvious. However, since in both groups sexual control is never enough and the satisfaction is so short lived, the danger is that the only ultimate and total control is *murder* — and this progression can and does take place. Many rapists that we have treated confess that as the sexually assaultive behavior progresses, the fantasies become more and more violent and eventually contain murder elements. Some sex offenders had actually reached this point prior to capture and had gotten away with one or more rape murders that remained unsolved. These *confessions* become a serious moral and ethical problem for the therapist treating sex offenders and cannot be predicted by testing or any other type of screening procedure. The ways in which we have dealt with this problem will be discussed in Chapter 19.

The issue of control also becomes a serious problem in fighting therapy resistance. The sex offender is constantly in a battle with the therapist for control of the session, what is disclosed, the speed of therapy and every other aspect of the overall treatment process. Learning to identify a particular offender's control needs and mechanisms is an important treatment consideration that needs to be addressed early in the treatment process. Let us look at a particular case that illustrates this type of control and it's source:

☐ BOBBY *is handsome and intelligent; he is employed successfully as an engineer. His arrest for a brutal rape shocks his family, the neighborhood, his fiancee and everyone at work and at the gym where he works out. Everyone unanimously believes that it is a case of mistaken identity. It is not.*

Bobby came from a home with a sadistically strict father and a passive, submissive mother. He had an older brother and a younger sister, with whom he got along well. For reasons never determined to this day, his father (now deceased) treated him worse than all of the other family members. Bobby's father was an alcoholic and when drunk he literally turned into a Jekyll and Hyde monster. His focus always centered on Bobby, whom he beat sadistically for the slightest provocation. The extent of the sadistic treatment can be demonstrated in the following example:

Bobby had forgotten to take out the garbage before going to school. When he came home, his drunken father beat him, made him undress naked, put a chain on him and tied him in one of the outdoor dog kennels (his father raised and sold pedigreed dogs). Bobby was forced to eat the same food the animals ate. He looked for help from his mother (whom he saw standing in an upstairs window looking at him with tears in her eyes) but none ever came. Out of intense fear, she did nothing to interfere with the father's sadistic treatment. His sister also watched from her bedroom window but never said a word.

This was only one of the sadistic treatments he received from his father until one day Bobby stood up to him and threatened to kill his father if he ever touched him again. From that day on, his father ignored him and never again touched Bobby.

In therapy, the focus at first was on his anger toward his father and anyone, including the therapist, who reminded him of his father. It took more than a year and a half of denial before Bobby was able to even consider that his anger was more towards his mother for not protecting and defending him, and that it was this anger that he projected onto his victims, nearly killing them during the rapes in uncontrollable rage.

Once this rage was thoroughly made conscious and ventilated, immediate behavioral changes were observed by everyone connected to Bobby. His therapeutic progress accelerated until, after another year, he was considered to be safe for return to the community.

RAGE-TRIGGERING TECHNIQUES

For some sexually assaultive personalities, none of the standard methods of ventilating their rage are effective. Their resistance is so great that special methods must be employed to achieve this important goal.

One of the methods that we have used successfully involves marathon therapy sessions and specialized badgering techniques. What occurs as a result, is a regression to earlier age levels and an actual reliving of past traumatic experiences. This is accompanied by hysterical conversion reactions that result in bleeding, pain, bruises and physical symptomology that, when examined by medical personnel may bring diagnoses that: "the trauma just occurred in the last hour or so." [*Note 1*]

NOTE

1. This technique is well-illustrated in an NBC-TV Movie [1980] entitled "Rage," based on a compilation of cases treated by this writer at the Adult Diagnostic & Treatment Center, Avenel — and strongly reminiscent of the case of *Joey* discussed in Chapter 13 — for which I served as consultant to the writer and technical director during filming on location and in Hollywood. For other specialized techniques, the reader is referred to the chapters on treatment.

5

Pervasive Guilt and Subjective Judgment

If one were to state that *guilt is the most destructive force in the universe,* one would be especially referring to the pervasive guilt of the sex offender. Differentiating between guilt and responsibility remains an important distinction in sex offender therapy that is often overlooked when dealing with resistance to change and/or "letting go" problems.

The guilt of the sex offender is not only exaggerated in degree, but is attributed to a range of actions from the immediate offense all the way back to being born. Not infrequently have we heard memories of childhood that contained hurtful remarks of parents that were never forgotten. These damaging and imprinting remarks can all be placed under the most damaging statement of all: *"I wish you had never been born!"*

Almost equal in frequency is the memory of hearing parents discuss their problems with the child and admitting that he had not been a planned child but an "accident" that either one or both parents regretted. With his inadequate personality, a weak and defective ego structure, and his already negative self-image, either type of statement is devastating to the child. Even if the event is repressed, the effects are the same: More reason for the child to hate himself and feel exaggerated guilt for the slightest failure, misbehavior or disappointment he inflicts upon his already rejecting parents.

Once learned and internalized, the offender uses the same ruler on himself all through growing up and into adulthood. Whatever he tries, he already has two strikes against him and considering his fear of failure, it is easy to see how all he can remember is failure after failure. Even an acknowledged success is mitigated by these feelings and cannot possibly balance the already overloaded scales of negative factors that he has accumulated over the years. Finding ways for him to succeed and accept the positive rewards for his success is a long and difficult task, not only for the therapist but also for the treatment team.

Since this guilt is all-pervasive, it affects every aspect of his existence: cognitive and behavioral, physical and athletic, educational and artistic, social and personal, moral and religious. Thus, the need for a *holistic* approach in the treatment planning (see Chapter 15.)

RULERS AND SUBJECTIVE JUDGMENT MEMORIES

One of the traits that is most resistant to change found in all sex offenders is the use of two rulers: one from the past (usually belonging to or learned from one of their parents) and one from their present adult self. I call these *subjective judgment memories,* and they always produce an irrational form of guilt!

The following schematic presents a summary of the factors involved in this phenomenon.

Hypocritically, sex offenders continue for years on end to use their ruler on friends, associates and even strangers that they do not particularly like. However, in all judgmental instances where they evaluate or analyze their own behavior, thinking or personality they use the ruler from childhood that is at least twice as large and demanding: the *subjective judgment memory ruler.*

In Chapter 2, where we discussed the inadequate personality structure of the sex offender, it was stated that if the individual scored a 90% in a test and this was the highest score in the

> **● A SCHEMATIC REPRESENTATION OF UNRESOLVED GUILT PROBLEMS AND THEIR CONSEQUENCES: SUBJECTIVE JUDGMENT MEMORIES**
>
> ☐ *Subjective judgment memory: A value judgment about a past behavior based on parental or authority values [rulers] that are not the values of the present child/adult.*
>
> ☐ *Perfectionism develops — failure is assured*
>
> ☐ *Self-punishing behavior results and affects motivation*
>
> ☐ *Severe guilt persists and affects all aspects of life*
>
> ☐ *The same behavior in others is considered acceptable*

classroom, it would still "not be good enough." When praised for the accomplishment the response would be something like: "It should have been 100%." The problem, however, is that, were it a 100%, then in keeping with the trait his response would be: "The test was too easy." In this no-win situation, the sex offender appears driven to see himself in a negative light and refuses to permit a positive interpretation or evaluation of his works or actions.

In interviewing and treating thousands of these individuals, the common theme of parents who could never be satisfied occurred over and over. No matter how hard he tried, and try he did, there was never any praise or reward for the child, and since acceptance and love were dependent on pleasing the parent(s), hurt, rejection and ultimately self- blame occurred.

In discussing this with one 27-year-old male offender (incarcerated for a series of some 60 rapes before he was caught) Kevin stated: *"It would be difficult to give up their (parents) rulers if I felt doing so would cause me to lose them and end up feeling alone."* When Kevin was asked how this translated into later life, he replied: "I'll only be loved and accepted if I am what he (the father) wanted me to be. In other words, live by his rulers. This didn't just apply to my father, it applied to every relationship I ever had until recently and even [in] the recent ones, it's there in certain areas — most importantly the emotional ones." Here, as in other areas already discussed and areas yet to come, insight is excellent and no change occurs.

Throughout these discussions, the inadequacy of insight as a solitary goal in sex offender treatment will be stressed continually. While it does answer many questions for the offender and *explains* much of the causality of the behaviors, *insight alone has never, in my experience, produced a single change.* This is quite a strong and potentially controversial statement that will need to be demonstrated over and over again, in case after case.

Another factor associated with using the two rulers is that of resulting perfectionism. As the child who earned the 100% grade on a test was dissatisfied, feeling that he should have done more, so the offender. A major treatment objective is to change the negative self-image of the sex offender. His trend toward perfectionism, however, prevents this goal from being achieved. Rational methods fail in this endeavor and it becomes apparent quite early in therapy that only the offender himself can change this condition by utter destruction of the parent-imposed ruler.

The irrationality and illogic of this condition needs further clarification by way of an example.

TODD'S BIG SECRET AND HIS USE OF HIS RULER

☐ *After many years of both group and individual therapy,* TODD, *with a great deal of hesitation and obvious pain, related to his group (15 mixed offender types) that during his very lonely and isolated early adolescent years, he had first masturbated his dog and then eventually taught the dog to mount and sodomize him. As happens in groups of this type who have been together for many years, several other group members (six or seven) admitted to similar sexual experiences with their dogs. Following their confessions, there was a great deal of emotional release with what appeared to the therapist to result in a successful session with much gained by all.*

Todd had appeared calm, talked openly about his feelings and expressed appropriate empathy and compassion for his fellow group members who had also "confessed" to this terrible sin. That evening, however, in an emergency individual therapy session that he requested, Todd told me that he still felt that what he had done was "sick, disgusting, unforgivable, sinful and rotten."

Nothing I tried worked, and while Todd was happy for the others who had obviously gained from the experience, his guilt had increased. He then decided that he would quit therapy and finish the 20 months he had to do on his sentence. No matter what approach was tried by several therapists and all of his friends, both in and out of the group, he never returned to therapy. A short six months following his release, he was caught in the act of attempting to rape a handicapped woman in her home and is now serving a heavy sentence in one of the state's prisons, not in the treatment center.

Todd is only one of many failures where the therapist has been unable to break the original ruler, although his own ruler that is used on everyone else but never on himself is positive and forgiving.

□ MARK, *after many years of therapy (approximately 12), and after hearing another group member discuss his ruler problem requested an individual session. After much hemming and hawing and a great deal of obvious distress, he stated that in all the years of his therapy he had hidden one deep, dark secret that was producing a large amount of irreconcilable guilt. After much encouragement, he told the therapist the following:*

From about the age of 11 or 12, he began peeping on his mother either when she was undressing or when she was in the bathroom. He would become sexually aroused and masturbate, either on the spot or back in his room. As the peeping episodes increased, he developed the fantasy of having intercourse with his mother and, in the fantasy, they both enjoyed the experience. Eventually he would replace his father in her life and especially in her bed.

The guilt from this experience had never been resolved and, even in the present time frame, when very lonely and/or depressed, he would revert to this forbidden fantasy, masturbate and then experience incredible guilt for weeks at a time, even to the degree of contemplating suicide. When he recovered emotionally to some extent, he was asked when he felt he could discuss this in his group and, as with Todd, his reply was that he would rather max-out (complete his sentence) without therapy (some 15 more years).

The astonishing thing about Mark's reaction was that, in his group, there were several other individuals who had "confessed" to the same or similar fantasies. His best friend in the institution had actually been involved sexually with his mother for several years during his adolescence and later adult, married life. Mark saw no problem with understanding, accepting, sympathizing, and being compassionate with his friend and never considered becoming judgmental with him or dissolving their relationship. Where his own peeping/fantasy behavior was concerned it was judgmentally labeled "perverted, disgusting, unforgivable, and sure to result in condemnation and rejection by the group."

When a sex offender verbalizes these contradictory, irrational values and concepts at the same time, in the same conversation, and agrees that it does not make sense, we can easily see the depth and extent of the problem. Where Mark was concerned, a year of intense individual therapy followed this confession with absolutely no change in behavior, attitude or value system. The original parent-child instilled ruler remained intact.

Where Kevin (mentioned several times earlier) was concerned, his dual desire to be a girl and have sex with his father (he had witnessed his father and his sister having sex in the nude) resulted in a ruler that measured him to be a "pervert, unnatural, sinful, bad," etc. The resulting guilt remained from age six or seven, when all of this began, until his present age 27, with, if anything, an increase in degree rather than any decrease or resolution.

Kevin used these memories to punish himself whenever he did not live up to one of his many perfectionistic standards. In contrast to the other cases mentioned, he brought his secret to group to cause rejection and degradation, which never occurred. In his mind, however, he would read into group members facial expressions or using his own "crystal ball" would put feelings and thoughts into the group members minds, actions toward him, etc. This continued for over ten years of treatment and only recently has begun to be resolved to a limited extent.

GUILT AS A BLOCK TO THERAPEUTIC PROGRESS

It is safe to state that guilt prevents any permanent or meaningful therapeutic progress since progress would be an ego positive and self-esteem enhancing occurrence. The individual with pervasive guilt does not deserve success of any kind nor behaviors that would be seen by others as well as himself as positive. Until the guilt is permanently identified, ventilated and (most importantly) *let go of* the client will not permit positive feedback from anyone including himself. If the therapist errs, at this point the results can be disastrous (not hyperbole!). An example will clarify:

☐ RUDY *arrived at the treatment center in a state of remission from a severe catatonic-schizophrenic episode (manifest by mannequin-like poses and behavior when frightened). The other offenders were very supportive and made Rudy feel safe and comfortable. Little by little, Rudy began to make friends and, after more than eight months of therapy, began to say a few words during his primary group. He even took the floor one time and did well, for a first experience.*

From one of his friends, it was learned that he had some background in electronics and that he was interested in working in the Video-Studio-Complex. After some time (almost a year) he became really good at editing videotape, a difficult and tedious task. Believing it would be a positive reinforcement, I went out of my way to meet Rudy in the control booth where he worked and to compliment him on what a terrific job he was doing. I said: "Keep this up and someday you could be the head of the Studio Complex!" Rudy said nothing and simply continued to do his work.

The following morning when I arrived at work, I was informed that there had been a problem in the main studio control booth and when I entered the booth I was informed that there had been some $5,000 worth of damage done to the videotape recorders. Someone had deliberately destroyed the recording heads and put the equipment out of alignment (a very serious and costly repair problem). Rudy arrived at work on time and when asked what he knew about the damage confessed to being the culprit, without explanation. As he was being led away to lock up (punishment cells), he stopped, turned around and said to me: "Now tell me how good I'm doing and what a great Studio Director I would make!"

Needless to say, I learned an important and quite expensive lesson. Positive feedback, while the client is still in his negative self-image stance, especially when guilt is the cause, will produce poor to tragic results, including regressive behaviors and even suicide attempts. There are also times when a client will quit therapy due to positive feedback occurring too soon or too strongly while he feels undeserving. It is therefore essential to carefully evaluate the progress a client is making and to assess exactly where he is at any given point in his therapy before taking the risk of making any positive comments.

This is also not the time to insist on risk-taking behaviors. All concentration must be focused on the source of the guilt and its elimination to a degree that makes positive feedback palatable. Thus, once again, we can see the importance of the need to assess readiness.

MARK AND SUBJECTIVE JUDGMENT

A constant frustration in therapy with the sex offender is a seeming double standard. An example at this point will clarify the problem:

> *After many years of therapy and a great deal of guilt, Mark finally admitted to masturbation fantasies, both in childhood and in the present, of having sex with his mother. Although he painfully related this in individual therapy, the therapist was unable to convince Mark to bring this to his group. The subjective judgment factor was present here in that several other members of Mark's group had already discussed the same fantasy and Mark was supportive, understanding and helpful to them. While it was all right for them to have sexual fantasies about their mothers, it was absolutely "disgusting, filthy and unforgivable" for Mark to have the same fantasy.*

The subjective judgment phenomenon is a constant and persistent barrier to letting go of either the past or present guilt that sex offenders, like Mark, experience and that prevents them from progressing in therapy.

Quite often, with compulsive sex offenders, when progress appears to be impeded and no visible or current explanation exists, the phenomenon of subjective judgment memories may be (and usually is) the problem.

Subjective judgment here refers to a judgment based on a personal value reaction which, in turn, is based on a value learned somewhere from birth to the time of the occurrence. The distinguishing characteristic of these judgments is that they do not apply to anyone else, only to the individual himself.

The sources of these learned value systems include: parents, relatives, school, religion, law, t.v./movies and any other childhood influence. Then, in adolescence, the source becomes the individual's peers.

HARRY AND THE ELEPHANT

Basically, what appears to occur in this phenomenon is that the adult, remembering an event or traumatic occurrence, is unable to separate his present value system from that of the child who, at a specific age, experienced the event or traumatic occurrence and then reacted to it judgmentally, usually in a negative manner. An example that clearly demonstrates this phenomenon follows:

☐ HARRY *is a 29-year-old violent rapist, highly motivated for therapeutic involvement and change. During his first interview and subsequently in one of his first group therapy sessions with 15 other offenders, he was able to openly discuss the offense for which he was incarcerated.*

Late one evening, in a popular park in his home town, Harry hid in wait and eventually grabbed a female jogger, pulling her into the brush. He viciously beat her while calling her every derogatory and filthy name he could think of, then ripped off her clothing and violently raped her, trying to hurt her as much as he could with his penis. Unsatisfied after his orgasm and continuing to deride and humiliate her, he then sodomized her, again trying to inflict as much pain with his penis weapon as possible. Following his second orgasm and still unsatisfied, he sat on her chest and made her lick the feces from his penis while continuing his verbal onslaught. Only then did he feel he had accomplished his goal and quickly left. The woman passed into unconsciousness and when found the next morning needed to be hospitalized. Following medical treatment for a week or more, she was transferred to a private psychiatric facility where she remains in treatment to this day.

Harry was able, although with some shame and guilt, to relate this story without apparent fear of rejection from his peers. Therapy for Harry progressed at a steady rate, but the primary therapist assigned to the case continued to feel that there was something wrong in the speed of Harry's progress. Harry, during the next five or six years, continued to grow and mature but never seemed quite ready for release to the community as safe.

In his sixth year of therapy, Harry requested an individual interview with the therapist and quite sheepishly and ashamedly stated that he had not been fair to the therapist since he had hidden a secret. He then went on, head down, to relate the following: One summer when Harry was 11 years old, he spent the summer working with an uncle who was a zookeeper. While very lonely, having no friends to play with, he became friends with a male elephant that he cleaned and cared for. He would spend all of his free time grooming and talking to the elephant. One day, in an aroused sexual state, he began to masturbate. The elephant watched and then came over and began to fondle Harry's genitals with his trunk. Harry noticed that the elephant had an erection and, on impulse, reached down and masturbated the elephant.

As his story ended, Harry was crying and hiding his face with his hands. The therapist then asked why he felt this badly about something that had happened 18 years before and Harry, vehemently stated: "That was the dirtiest, filthiest, sickest and most disgusting thing that anyone could possibly do."

The therapist then asked when Harry planned to bring this story to his group, and Harry responded angrily, almost shouting, that he would never tell this story to anyone else, ever again. If that meant his doing the rest of his sentence (14 years remaining), he would refuse further therapy and do the 14 years.

It appears unreasonable to believe that the 29-year-old adult who was able to relate the story of the violent and vicious rape would have a value system that would not allow him to face his peers with the story of an event that occurred when he was 11 years old. To confirm this hypothesis, Harry was asked to imagine being in group and hearing this story told by his closest friend, Bob. When asked how he would react and what he would say to Bob or feel about what Bob had done, Harry became his usual sensitive, empathetic self, stating he would have felt sorry for the young boy who was that lonely and desperate. In regard to the adult Bob, it would make no difference in their friendship nor would he feel any of the disgust he felt about his own 11-year-old self.

What appears to occur in these instances is a dual value system: one that existed at the time of the event/trauma and one that exists today in the now adult person. As is true in other areas with sex offenders, the inability to let go occurs here as well.

When a disguised version of the story was told in his group the following week, more than 90% of the group admitted by a show of hands that they also were hiding a subjective judgment memory but not one of them would share the memory with group members. Several wrote to the therapist and offered to relate the memory privately as long as it would remain confidential from their peer group.

Several more groups were canvassed with the same result, including an aftercare group of released offenders in the community. Here again, while not one of them would share the memory in a group setting, several volunteered, *in fact requested* to discuss the memory in private with the assurance that no one would ever find out.

The range of these subjective judgment memories appears unlimited and includes:

- masturbation fantasies of sex with mothers,
- religiously prohibited behaviors,
- a great deal of animal sex,
- involvement with urine and feces, and
- murder.

Here, again, as in other areas of the sex offender personality, this information would never come to light unless the therapist, in some directive fashion, asks the right questions or suggests the importance of the child's maintaining control of the adult's mind.

JUDGMENT VERSUS CURIOSITY

When dealing with the subjective judgment memories phenomenon, a new theory/hypothesis became necessary. As in all other areas involving treatment of the repetitive compulsive sex offender, a concrete and graphic method and/or explanation had

---

• CONSEQUENCES OF JUDGMENTALISM IN ASSESSING EVENTS OF ONE'S PAST LIFE

- *1) Guilt and the attending emotions.*
- *2) Feelings of being:*
  - → *Inferior,*
  - → *different,*
  - → *sick/perverted,*
  - → *abnormal,*
  - → *relationally unacceptable.*
- *3) Isolation.*
- *4) Distrust of self and others.*
- *5) Fear of rejection.*
- *6) Depression (from mild to suicidal).*
- *7) Activation of the classic defense mechanisms especially: denial, minimization, projection, externalization; and, if the trauma is severe enough, repression.*

to be used. In dealing with this problem, it was postulated that *judgment stops all therapeutic progress.*

Thus, whenever a client goes into a judgmental mode, it is easy to see why little or no therapeutic progress occurs, even after several years. In my experience, I have had sex offenders in this mode for as much as 12 years, especially where there was an unrevealed subjective judgment memory involved. The therapist, with either the offender or the victim, must stop this practice as early in the treatment process as possible. In contrast, *curiosity* or the "I wonder why?" approach opens all doors to therapeutic progress on a very rapid and ego satisfying level.

In order for the curiosity approach to work, the patient must be taught *distancing* techniques. The simplest method of accomplishing this is to promulgate and insist on the "I'm no longer that person" perception. An easy method that has worked successfully for me, both with adults and children, is to use a different name for the child who experienced the trauma. It is best to ask the patient the nickname he was given by parents and friends and answered to as a child (Billy for Bill, Red for John, etc.). If he still uses that nickname, then the client is asked to pick a name he now feels suits the little child he was. When this is done, the chosen name often reveals a great deal about how the patient feels about his past self. Names such as "The Jerk," "Fuck- up," "Stinky," "Thing," "Fatso," and other derogatory choices all reflect the persistence of negative feelings about the child within. In the "Now" technique (see Chapter 18), the patient refers to the person in the mirror as *you* rather than *I* to effect this necessary distancing. Once distancing is effected, the patient can (1) become more objective, analytical, or empathetic, or make connections to developmental behavior or to present problem focus, *or* (2) effect a "makes sense" conclusion.

6

Relational Issues

The next characteristic to consider in our long list is the sex offender's inability to be assertive. He remains and has been for most of his life either *passive* or *aggressive.*

Whenever I do training with teachers and school administrators on this subject, I ask the fifth grade teacher in the audience to raise her/his hand and then ask them to think about two boys in their classroom who never play or associate with their classmates (peers). I then suggest that one will go to the third grade boys where he will become the *leader* since he is older, stronger, appears to know more and can easily control third graders. This is the *deny-er* (more about him later). The other boy goes to seventh and eighth graders where he becomes the *mascot.* He never has to compete with them but can become the bat boy or locker room towel boy and receive protection, acceptance, travel with the teams, even wear a letter of the team, yet have to give little or nothing in return. This is the *accept-er* (more about him later, also). The teachers are able to immediately think of the names of boys in their class who fit the above description.

Most sex offenders fall into one of the two categories above: *accept-ers* or *deny-ers.* What appears to happen is the basis for the theoretical framework upon which our treatment techniques are based: As children, sex offenders appear to have been basically inadequate personalities as described above (see characteristic *inadequate personality*, Chapter 2). Part of this lifelong adjustment pattern is a fear of any emotionally laden situation, especially if confrontation is a part of it. The overall effect is either a totally *passive* (wimpy) manner in dealing with everyone, especially authority figures or peers from whom they perceived threat/danger, or a totally *aggressive* manner in dealing with situations. The aggression can either be verbal or physical, or often both. It is easy to see, then, how the former go to children with whom they feel safe and *in control*. The latter use their aggression on everyone to constantly maintain control.

Control then becomes a major issue in all dealings with the sex offenders, as we saw in Chapter 4 with the case of Bobby. Whether the control is used by the *deny-er* or the *accept-er*, it will always be there and it must work in order for any satisfaction from the behavior to be realized. Even the flasher (exhibitionist) exerts control in his act. Try not to look when he flashes; it is literally impossible. Once the intended victim does look, a smile covers his face that says *"Gotcha!"*

For the pedophiles and hebophiles, getting the child to cooperate in their seduction, no matter how minor, provides the same control-produced satisfaction. Remember HOWIE (whose case is discussed in Chapters 2, 9, and 12), the compulsive pedophile who was so frightened that he never actually touched his victims? Howie's control came from the fact that, without saying a word, his smile alone told the children what pleased him and how they could get his acceptance. He was able to get them to pose nude and also to pose nude with erections, although he had never discussed sex with them. He was a master manipulator who, with a smile and a "My, my!" or "Wonderful!" was able to teach the boys what he wanted and how they could get invited on another weekend nature/camping trip. Not only did this satisfy Howie's control needs but also assuaged his highly punitive conscience. He easily rationalized that "the boys were only doing what they wanted and posing in the manner they chose."

Thus Howie excused himself from all responsibility and guilt. Throughout his interrupted treatment, he never actually accepted blame or guilt for what he had done, nor did he ever agree that his behavior was damaging to the children.

In sexually assaultive behavior, the control elements are more than obvious and are often more important than the sexual gratification. In fact there have been many cases of attempted rape where, once the submission and total control are accomplished, the sexually assaultive person (S.A.P.) leaves and does not complete the rape itself.

MORE EVIDENCE OF THE IMPORTANCE OF THE CONTROL ISSUE.

Harry, a violent rapist, (whose case was discussed in Chapter 5) needed *absolute control* in order to achieve any satisfaction from his rapes. If he suspected either that the victim was enjoying the act (pelvic movement, moans, etc.) or that he was not producing enough pain, he would perform other acts that he made sure were painful. When he was finished, his last sadistic act was to force the victim to say that she enjoyed what he had done and that he was a great lover (under threat of further violence and/or harm).

Bobby (see Chapter 4) on the other hand, could stop himself from going any further once he felt in complete control. Once he had the victim undressed, he was exposed and erect and felt that he had achieved the control element in the rape, he would tell the victim to get dressed and would run away. If, at that point, he did not feel that control had been reached, he would complete the rape. If after the rape, he *still* did not feel that control had been reached, he would do something more until he reached that point of *absolute control.*

Each sex offender develops his own control method. These methods are as varied and different as are the offenders themselves. Pedophiles, for example, feel *absolute control* when they manipulate the child into initiating the sex, at least one time with no hint or suggestion from the offender. To them, this equals conquest and proves their superiority and mastery over the victim. As further examples are presented, this control need, especially in the relationships of the offender, will be clearly seen, regardless of the issue being discussed.

SEVERELY IMPAIRED INTERPERSONAL RELATIONSHIPS

An often missed characteristic of the repetitive compulsive sex offender is that, while he may and often does appear to be quite a sociable person, the fact is that he relates only on a *surface* plane. He never really becomes intimate or involved with anyone, even his wife or closest friend. His inability to trust and/or to become vulnerable persists throughout his life, especially if he was sexually molested or traumatized as a child and never resolved it. While he desperately wants acceptance and closeness, he is unwilling to risk being hurt and thus maintains a *distance* in all his relationships. Should the other person involved appear to be getting too close, he will push the person away in any manner he can, even to the point of deliberately destroying the relationship. *Safety* becomes paramount in all his dealings with other people and he will choose loneliness rather than risk any further chance of being hurt, betrayed or rejected — the fears that control his behavior daily.

It is easy to see, therefore, why the repetitive compulsive sex offender becomes involved with so many victims. Even the pedophiles and hebophiles rarely have only one victim. Here, as in his adult relationships, the fears remain and, as soon as he feels himself getting too close, he pushes away and rejects before being rejected.

Frequently, due to this *vulnerability fear*, the repetitive compulsive sex offender will say that no matter how hard he tries in a relationship he gets rejected. It often takes quite a long time to get him to see that in some subtle way he destroyed the relationship. An example will clarify:

☐ *Kevin (whose case is discussed in Chapters 3 and 5) has gone through this cycle literally hundreds of times. In each instance, he truly and sincerely wants the relationship and all starts out well. Then, in an almost paranoidal cycle, he begins to set the other person up by putting expectations and demands on the individual that no one would allow. A single missed phone call, an item missing in a gift package, a disagreement over even the most trivial factor, and the process begins. A record of these occurrences is kept and each one adds to the proof that either the individual is not sincere with him or in some way plans to use him. It is impossible to show Kevin that, in reality, it is he who is using the other person or that his expectations are unrealistic and/or inappropriate. Unconsciously, Kevin wants to believe the worst since only separatton or loss of the relationship will bring him back to his needed state of safety. The pain, hurt and sorrow he feels when the relationship ends are prices he is willing to pay (or so he says). Until he no longer is willing to pay so high a price, no change will occur.*

THE SEX OFFENDER'S INABILITY TO RELATE TO PEERS

As early as the lower grades of grammar school, this factor can be detected and a referral made before it's too late. The inadequate personality that may or may not evolve into a sex offender personality cannot, even at very early ages, relate to his peer group. As stated above, what usually occurs is that he becomes either a leader or mascot in relation to other children in his younger years and to adults as he grows older. Which type he becomes is dependent on his ego strength, his self-esteem and his ability to deal with his inadequacy.

For both types of boys, this coping mechanism works through grammar school and before puberty. But once puberty is reached and the all important psychological shifts occur, especially that of wanting to please peers rather than wanting to please adults, a crisis occurs that changes and affects the remainder of his life if not detected and treated. Being *different* now becomes his primary preoccupation and the negative judgments occur in rapid succession. Selective perception runs rampant.

Two examples will clarify the concept:

☐ DENNIS *(an accept-er) has never felt that he was like other children his age, beginning at his earliest memory, age five to six. No reasons can be elicited from Dennis but if pushed he will use terms like "sissy, fraidy cat, nerd, weirdo, etc." while looking at the floor and being obviously upset and appearing depressed. When he enters grammar school, the situation worsens and he becomes both an object of ridicule and a punching bag for the older boys. He increases his isolation, running home immediately after school or watching other children play from a safe distance.*

High school and the onset of puberty produces depression close to suicidal levels. He literally sticks out like a sore thumb, simply attending school, sitting in the back of the room, never volunteering to answer questions, and if picked to participate by the teacher, standing, head down and silent until released. College produces changes in that he is accepted in a fraternity where he becomes a slave to his fraternity brothers and an even further object of laughter and ridicule. One evening, as the brothers were drinking beer on the fraternity house porch, the fraternity president, drunk and in a nasty mood, walks over to Dennis, unzips and urinates on him as the other brothers laugh hysterically. Dennis sits there through the incident, saying nothing and feeling that this is a price he must pay for his membership in the fraternity since he certainly doesn't deserve it. Being used as a chauffeur, lending money that is never returned, doing laundry, buying tickets for sports events, paying checks at restaurants, etc., all continue as payments to the present time.

After a year or more of therapy, Dennis could admit to the reality of his being used and that these were not his true friends but retorted, "If I give this up, there will be nothing and no one in my life! It's better than nothing!"

Until Dennis' self-image and self-esteem improve, his life will remain the same, that of a true nerd and wimp, being taken advantage of by anyone for the illusion that they are his friend. Guilt prevents any change from occurring and, to date, we have been unable to uncover the source of the guilt.

☐ KEN *(a deny-er), on the other hand, has been a sociable, popular child from his earliest years and the favorite of both his parents. From his first days at school, he was popular and liked by his peers, the teachers and the staff as well. He was always a success at anything he did and appeared quite happy in his life. At age 14, he committed his first rape but convinced the victim that no one would believe her since she was unpopular and not really liked by anyone. She agreed and left the school instead.*

The rapes continued until he was finally caught and sent to the treatment unit at age 31. Again the pattern continued: he became a leader in everything, including his therapy group, was the most popular man in the unit, was given the best and most trusted job in the institution and prospered. Within two years (of a 30 year indeterminate sentence) he earned entrance into the parole process. This meant that he was approved and recommended by his primary therapist, a group of therapists serving as an examining board, and a civilian review board from the community, all before even seeing the State Parole Board who also unanimously approved his parole.

Fewer than four months back in the community, he visited me one night in the hospital where I was undergoing some tests for a possible ulcer (a perk of prison work!) and asked me for a recommendation to graduate school where he hoped to become a psychologist and work with children of sexual abuse. I was thrilled and happily signed the forms.

At the end of visiting hours he left, promising to see me the following week. Driving out of the parking lot with a large number of other visitors, Ken was behind a pretty young lady in a convertible and, without thought or planning followed her a short distance as she drove behind an apartment complex into her garage. When she shut the engine of her car off, Ken entered the convertible, robbed her of her jewelry and raped her.

All of this occurred fewer than 30 minutes after his visit to my room. It should also be noted that he was engaged to be married at the time. In less than an hour, I was awakened by a supervising nurse and informed that two local detectives wanted to see me. They told me what happened and then related that after the rape, Ken walked down a main highway toward the police station. Ken knew where he was and where the police station was located. He easily could have gotten away by driving in the opposite direction toward a major interstate highway since the victim had not seen his car. Once back in the treatment unit as a parole violator waiting for his new rape charge to be processed, Ken, crying and depressed, finally told me that he had never believed that other people really knew who he was or liked the real Ken, only the social image he portrayed and the actor he had been all of his life. The reasons for Ken's self-hatred were never uncovered and, after a few months and his new sentence, he again became the actor.

A therapist who specialized in classical behavior modification techniques took over the case (I wisely withdrew since I had been completely fooled the first time) and within a short period of time, Ken was once again paroled as "cured." This time, the therapy for his *rape problem* worked.

THE DANGERS OF SYMPTOM REMOVAL

As a result of Ken's behavior, we quickly learned the dangers of *symptom removal.* In just under six months, Ken was rearrested and is now serving a life sentence for conspiracy to murder his wealthy uncle, whom he felt was humiliating, berating and depriving his mother of her true inheritance (his own delusions according to his mother).

Deny-ers are the most difficult type of sex offender to work with and to assess for real or true change. While Ken was a very dramatic failure, he was only one of many of this type for whom therapy was never effective until new techniques were finally developed that do work with *deny-ers.* These techniques will be discussed in Chapters 9 through 19 inclusive.

REPRESSION AND TRAUMA INDUCED COMPULSION

Many of the sex offenders that we have treated, complain of a driving compulsion that, no matter what they try, will not cease.

Dennis arrived at the office for his first interview, visibly upset, depressed and close to suicide. He could not look the therapist in the eye and related that he could no longer endure living with his problem. Slowly the following compulsion was described: Dennis goes out looking for young boys with their shirts off and with a slightly protruding stomach. They also must be thin, inadequate-looking and weaker than the other boys involved. He then fantasizes that one of the other boys is punching him in the stomach and this gives him an erection. He then quickly rushes home to his bedroom and fucks a towel with the fantasy getting more and more violent. Following his orgasm, he becomes grossly depressed and wants to die.

He also related the following facts: he is a virgin (has never had sex with any other human being) and has never masturbated with his hand; cannot masturbate to any other fantasy but the one above. Dennis also fails persistently at work and in all relationships. His "friends" all belong to his college fraternity and treat him like a "dip" (his term) making him a servant and degrading him publicly to the extent of urinating on him in front of the whole group.

Regardless of treatment modalities used, no real change occurs in over a year's involvement in therapy. His fantasy continues to increase in frequency as well as degree of pathology (recent fantasies include the victim being brutally murdered). There is no doubt in the therapist's mind that Dennis was sexually molested as a child and that some element of the molestation resulted in severe guilt that he is unable to expiate. Thus his self-destructive behavior.

He now realizes that his problems at work and in all of his relationships are self-induced and utilized to punish himself. When asked why, he does not consciously know the answer. In his dreams, more and more material has begun to emerge, including an incident in the park where he is taken away from his friends by an older man in dark clothing. The age is most probably seven, as all the children in the fantasy are age seven also.

While the age is known, the event remains *repressed* and, until we can break through the defensive barriers and bring the event back into consciousness, the compulsion will continue and unfortunately will also increase in both frequency and severity. A different type of case will clarify the concept.

MIKE: DEVIATION AND CONNECTION TO MOLESTATION AS A CHILD

☐ MIKE *was an advisor to a boys' group. He was employed as a lieutenant in the navy reserve, working toward a promotion to captain. Mike was married and had three young children, two girls, ages five and seven, and a new baby son, nine months old, named* TIMMY. *His wife,* JANE, *was a loving mother and good wife to Mike who reported "a good marriage with a wonderful husband who was caring and who doted on his children." Although they had always wanted a son, a serious change occurred in their lives when Timmy was born. Mike became more nervous, agitated and short-tempered than ever before and appeared to have lost his interest in sex, at least where his wife was concerned.*

Mike called for an appointment, indicating that he had a problem having sex with his wife and needed help. During the first interview, he related that while impotent with his wife almost all of the time, he was masturbating more and more with firm erections. He dated the onset of the problem with his wife's return home with their newborn son. It was obvious that Mike was not telling all. This was discussed as being a problem and barrier to my helping him. After protesting that this was not true and that he was being completely open, Mike became angry and abruptly ended the session without making another appointment.

Two weeks later, Mike called and made an appointment for the same evening. From the moment of his arrival, it was obvious that he was agitated, emotionally upset and frightened. I helped him to relax, telling him to take his time and to use his own words. Mike began to cry and slowly related that while helping his wife with the children by changing and bathing his son, Timmy, he was getting more and more interested in Timmy's penis and was having erections, just staring at it. He was also masturbating to thoughts of masturbating little Timmy and this frightened and disgusted him. He said he would rather die than molest his son or any of his children. He also related that this had never happened when he changed or bathed his two daughters.

Crying and sobbing for several minutes, Mike continued and related that on an overnight campout with a boys' group, he awoke in the middle of the night, noticed that one of the boys had kicked off his blankets (a boy he had been obsessed with for some time but in a non-sexual, paternalistic manner), went over to cover him and saw that he was exposed and had an erection. Without thinking, Mike masturbated the boy to orgasm and ejaculation. The boy did not appear to wake up (or pretended not to) and Mike was immediately filled with disgust and revulsion. That evening, when he returned home, he was arrested. This occurred just after the birth of his son and the bathing incident. At this point, I asked Mike if he really wanted to understand the problem and alleviate it. He insisted that he would do anything to have that happen. I then asked him to tell me about his own sexual molestation. He immediately began to deny it, saying it never happened to him and I simply kept asking the same question, over and over again, for the next 15 to 20 minutes. Suddenly, he sat up and yelled: "Oh, my God! It did happen! I remember!"

As a child, Mike was molested by a boarder his mother took in following his father's death. They had a mutual relationship for over two years and the roomer became the substitute father Mike never had and always wanted. The adult bought him clothes and other presents; took him on trips; showed him physical affection, (hugging, tousling hair, etc.) and became an idol. These were the happiest years that Mike could remember, since his own father was an alcoholic who died when Mike was only nine years old.

At the end of the two year period, the roomer disappeared and Mike felt abandoned, rejected, betrayed and used. Shortly after this, the family moved to another city where the grandparents lived. Mike made new friends who, discovering that he was an adolescent virgin, quickly remedied the situation. Mike began a heterosexual period that lasted through adolescence, into his marriage and up to the time that he molested the young boy.

The next few sessions were used to explore and ventilate this repressed memory fully. We began to explore the effects of the molestation and repressed trauma throughout Mike's life from the abandonment to the present.

Mike quickly perceived and understood the molestation of the boy on the camping trip. He was depressed at the time; was anxious and frightened by the idea of having a son but did not know why; was having problems with a superior at work; and, finally, had no real male friends, which he wanted but feared. The next hurdle was his conclusion that the memory of the two-year homosexual relationship with the roomer, coupled with his molestation of the boy on the camping trip and his attraction to his son Timmy's penis, all made him a queer and that he'd rather be dead. Sex education followed and Mike accepted the fact that he was bisexual, but that did not mean he had to act on it. Following the session where this acceptance took place, he was able to again have sex with his wife with no trace of the impotence.

EMOTIONS SUPPRESSED OR DISPLACED

Another extremely difficult area to work with in sex offender therapy is that of *emotions*. While some sex offenders can emote easily and spontaneously, others simply cannot show any emotion except anger. Even their anger release is minimal and overly controlled.

Tracing emotions back into childhood can be difficult if not dangerous. Repressed memories, usually containing one or more traumas of either a sexual or nonsexual nature, may take many years to uncover. Some of these memories are so deeply repressed that even hypnosis cannot break through the defensive barriers. When, and if, they break through, the amount and intensity of the accompanying rage is impossible to predict. Therefore precautions for the safety of the patient as well as the therapist must be prearranged.

Regression techniques are useful in dealing with this problem, but can be dangerous and require a great deal of training and experience before they are utilized. Complicating the entire area of emotions in the sex offender is a system of *defective values*, usually surrounding the concept of *manhood*. Since this is a highly sensitive area for sex offenders, the defective value system must be exposed and resolved, before any attempt to deal with the emotional constriction and suppression or repression. The *double standard* of the sex offender (see section on "rulers") applies and confuses matters more: one sex offender may be highly supportive of another sex offender who is emoting and even congratulate him on releasing the deep feelings that have been held in check for so long. However, when it comes to doing it himself, nothing happens. He intellectually verbalizes feelings of hurt, pain, disappointment and sorrow, but behaviorally nothing occurs.

Repression and all of its effects play a major role in blocked emotions. The more intellectual the individual involved, the harder to break through the barriers. Some of the sex offender's reasoning involved is valid: "If I allow myself to *feel*, I might remember what happened to me or what I did. Then, I'll either hurt terribly or have to feel guilty about what happened and I don't want to do either."

Here, again, Kevin comes to mind (his case was discussed in Chapters 3 and 5). After many, many years of therapy that produced major positive changes in Kevin's personality, he was still unable to spontaneously emote. He stated that he wanted to emote and felt emotions beginning, but then they were choked off. Concurrently, Kevin suspected that he had been molested, possibly by someone very close to him, but could not "remember" it happening. Each time this was discussed, he became visibly sad and depressed and looked like he was about to cry, but neither the memory nor the emotion ever surfaced. Every method possible, including hypnosis, failed, but there remained too many unanswered questions and unexplainable behaviors that could only have resulted from sexual trauma. For over ten years of combined therapy with several therapists and in many modalities, the search continued but was never successful.

Another method the sex offender uses to avoid dealing with emotions is *displacement*. Like a small child (which, emotionally, the sex offender often is) he projects/displaces the emotions or the reasons for his emotional reactions onto others:

- "He made me mad!" —
- "She hurt my feelings!" —
- "It wasn't my fault; if he had not gotten me angry I would not have hit him."

Getting the sex offender to accept responsibility for his own feelings and reactions is a difficult and long-term task. The use of "I" statements applies here, as will be discussed in Chapter 10. Maintaining a therapy rule, for both individual and group, that the offender must start all explanatory or judgmental sentences with the word "I" puts all the responsibility on him and usually prevents blame from being projected or displaced.

I often use the following example with clients to explain the above concept:

- *Wrong:* "She hurt my feelings when I asked her for a date and she rejected me." becomes:
- *Correct:* "I got hurt and felt rejected when I asked her for a date and she said no."

More on this later.

7

Sexual Performance Problems

STRONG PERFORMANCE NEEDS

Sex offenders, for the most part, have never had sex for fun. All of their sexual behavior, whether masturbatory or with another person, serves a purpose and that purpose, most of the time, is to make them feel better about themselves by either proving something or denying something.

THE SEX OFFENDER'S USE OF MASTURBATION

Masturbation, from the time it was first learned accidentally, discovered naturally or performed on them, carried a meaning other than pleasuring which immediately became *imprinted* (see Chapter 11). The most common self- learned masturbatory motive was to feel better when either rejected, punished, lonely or depressed in relation to a specific event.

☐ KEVIN *was the last of six children and was six years younger than his nearest sibling, a sister. Kevin was not a planned child and his arrival added an additional burden to an already burdened family. His father was a workaholic who was rarely at home and when home was always tired and not to be disturbed. From his earliest memories, Kevin felt alienated and rejected by most of his family, except his mother. He wanted acceptance from his father desperately but never received it. Usually, when he asked his father to help him with homework or some other task, his father was busy sleeping or reading the newspaper. He received similar rejection from his older siblings most of the time. Kevin thus spent a great deal of time alone in his attic room in fantasies of all types: from hero fantasies to anger revenge fantasies where he would punish the entire family.*

Rubbing against the mattress one day, he discovered the pleasant feelings it produced in his penis, and this became a ritual whenever he was alone. As he grew older, he began manipulating his penis with his hand and this replaced the mattress rubbing quite quickly. His masturbation pattern had developed and now, regardless of the negative occurrence, off to his room he would go to "make myself feel better." School problems and social difficulties were added to the list of reasons to masturbate and his frequency went from once or twice a day to five or six times a day. On a really bad day, he would masturbate a dozen times or more and the fantasies became more and more angry and punitive.

Even in adult life, when married, his compulsive masturbation continued, often after he had completed sex with his wife. Kevin cannot recall even one time that sex was for enjoyment only or when sex occurred when he was in a good or positive frame of mind. (More of Kevin throughout our discussions.)

☐ MARK *was ten years old when he was sexually molested by his older brother, whom he admired and from whom he desperately wanted acceptance. Prior to this occasion, he had no sexual knowledge and had not discovered masturbation. On a camping trip alone with his brother, Mark was talked into going skinny-dipping and then lying nude in the sun on the shore to dry off. Pleasantly tired and dozing off, he felt his brother move closer to him, begin rubbing his chest and stomach and then touch and fondle his penis. Frightened and pretending to be asleep, he allowed his brother to continue and when erect, his brother masturbated him to orgasm. Mark had never felt anything like this before and, although still scared and confused by his brother's behavior, he enjoyed the experience and said nothing. His brother then told him to stop faking since now it was his turn and placed Mark's hand on his penis and told him what to do. Some minutes later, fully aroused, his brother told him to turn over, got on top of him and without explanation penetrated him anally. While there was a great deal of initial pain, Mark soon found himself enjoying the sodomy and becoming highly aroused again himself. Very little was said and when his brother finished with him, Mark was told to go into the lake and wash himself and not to tell anyone what had occurred or he would never let him go anywhere with him again.*

Mark was extremely confused at this point: on the one hand, he intuitively felt that he had done something he should not have and that he didn't want anyone else to know about; on the other hand, he enjoyed being masturbated by his brother and also enjoyed his brother sodomizing him. However, his feelings about himself dramatically changed. Over the next few weeks and months, the brother's attention to Mark increased and besides giving him presents, the brother showed Mark all the affection he had always wanted from his father (who had deserted the family).

Mark's mother was ecstatic about his new and closer relationship with his brother and encouraged it as strongly as she could. As can be expected, the brother planned another camping trip only two weeks from the first and Mark somehow knew that it was time to pay for all the gifts and the attention. This time, the molestation took place at night when they were preparing for bed and the brother told Mark that he knew that Mark enjoyed what he had done to him. He also mentioned their new relationship and the gifts, attention, etc., and then (the brother was now naked and erect) asked Mark to play their game again. Mark's intuition of payment was now confirmed and since he desperately wanted the affection, love and presents, he agreed. Their games went on for several years, until one day the brother announced his engagement, much to Mark's shock and horror. By now his love for his brother was more than brotherly and Mark, needing the sex more than the brother did, had become the initiator. Mark went out looking for sex and a new brother and being a good-looking, slim and clean teenager, he had few problems in finding more than one adult to play the now lost role of his brother.

Sex now became a payment for love, affection and material gain in Mark's new and distorted value system. Mark was now a male prostitute and, no matter how hard he tried to rationalize his behavior, he realized it. All through these years, Mark understood that he was gay. Being gay, however, was a taboo with his mother, his friends and everyone he associated with except the adult males he was now servicing.

Self-image deteriorated and he often allowed painful or forced sodomy to be performed on him in order to punish himself for being abnormal. Finally, in a desperate attempt to salvage his manhood, he began dating girls with the hope that by having sex with them, he would be magically converted to heterosexuality. The problem was that all the time he was in bed with a woman, in order to perform he was fantasizing being with a male. Also, in his masturbatory behavior he was obsessed with inserting objects into his rectum to simulate being sodomized, which had now become an unwanted obsession. His self-hate and the blame he projected onto his mother, who should have protected him from his brother instead of encouraging their relationship, finally resulted in rape.

It is interesting to note that in all of his rapes, after intercourse was complete, he forcibly sodomized each victim. In fact, as the rapes continued, he eliminated vaginal sex and proceeded directly to the sodomy which he tried to make as painful as possible.

For similar reasons and based on the principle of *imprinting*, every sex offender that I have met and treated had some distorted sex value that remained from the first incident of sexual orgasm to the time of his offense. Some of these include the distorted values that *sex equals love, revenge, comfort, payment, an equalizer, manhood, acceptance,* or *a rite of passage.* All of these distorted values grossly affect the overall personality of the developing inadequate personality and add a sexual dimension that slowly but surely becomes *compulsive.*

First, an *obsession* with sex begins and may last throughout an entire childhood, adolescence and into adulthood. This was the case with Kevin. Playing with friends, his first school experiences and all social contacts were tainted by sexual obsession; this was followed by compulsive masturbation, graduating to exposing himself at every possible opportunity; finally, it ended in sexual molestation and sexual assault.

The direction of later behavior appears directly linked with the initial sexual experience. Both Kevin and Mark ended up as sexually assaultive persons but arrived there by totally different routes. Let us look at each *path* and the differences in the two boys' development from sexually abused children into rapists with multiple victims and severe blocking to all therapeutic effort.

Kevin's path, described above, hinged almost totally on his father's rejection. Why, then, did he not become sexually assaultive against males? The answer may lie in *where* the child places the blame for his condition. In the majority of young children, the mother figure is the protector and the one who should look out for all of the needs of the growing child — physical, protective, and emotional as well.

Females in Kevin's life were always his problem and the group on which he placed all blame for his condition:

- His father preferred his sisters, females, over him and showed them the love that Kevin wanted;

- His mother then showed more attention to the sisters than to Kevin and his brothers (who were independent and didn't need it).

- Since his mother rejected him, in Kevin's distorted thinking she also rejected his penis (his maleness).

- His mother used embarrassment to deal with his misbehaviors and this increased his rage and anger.

- His attempts to meet and date girls in school all ended up in rejection and humiliation (he acted like a nerd!).

- His wife was not pretty and did not satisfy him sexually. She did not accept his requests for deviant sexual acts, including "play rape" (his term) and bondage. He also suggested water sports but she refused.

- When he flashed girls and women, they laughed and made comments about his flaccid penis size (he wanted them to come over and fondle him and then offer themselves for sex).

From his earliest memories, there was an inordinate amount of anger toward women, with only two or three examples of anger towards males, mainly as a result of his brothers' rejection and his father's rejection as well.

His compulsive sexual needs, especially for fellatio as acceptance of his penis, were constantly thwarted by women. Then, in his first incarceration, he became entangled with an older man who introduced him to homosexuality (the older man fellated him regularly and finally fulfilled his need). Kevin developed an intense need to deny his homosexuality and to deny the fact that he now masturbated to fantasies of fellating other men in the treatment unit. Upon release, his need for sex with women became totally compulsive and his large number of rapes resulted.

Mark, on the other hand, developed a totally different path to his rape behavior:

- Mark was rejected from birth by his father. His mother was weak, alcoholic and non-supportive of his needs;

- At age ten, Mark was raped by his older brother who told him that he was *"better than any woman he had ever had."* From this experience, Mark developed strong doubts about his masculinity and suspected that he was feminine and gay.

- Mark never had any close friends and, after the rape by his brother, coincidentally, in his first incarceration as a juvenile became a *kid* (submissive younger male to an older inmate) for one of the older and stronger inmates who showed him concern, affection, caring and protection. In return, Mark became his *"woman"* and this further confirmed in his mind that there was something wrong within himself and that he was at fault for *seducing* his brother as well as his friend in prison.

- Mark blamed his mother for all of his problems: his poverty and lack of emotional support; his embarrassment over her drinking and bringing home men for the night; his rape by his brother that he was sure she condoned; and ultimately for not being the mother he wanted and saw at his other friends' homes.

- In attempting to deny that he was homosexual, he attempted to have sexual relationships with as many women as he could. However, after each affair he felt dissatisfied and used. None of the relationships lasted (he made sure of that!). He could not accept blame or responsibility and projected all blame for all of his problems on one or another woman in his life.

- Mark had a strong need to *destroy* the woman inside himself and he did this through his victims, although he was not conscious of that fact until years into therapy.

- He could not accept the concept of being bisexual and therefore had to prove his masculinity through heterosexual behavior, including rape.

- Being an abused child himself, whenever he saw a woman abusing children or animals, he became enraged and immediately chose her as his next possible victim. One woman he raped he had witnessed abusing her little dog in the backyard. He knew from that moment that he would *"get back at her his way!"*

As in the case of Kevin, Mark's self-hate and totally negative self-image were major barriers to therapeutic progress and did not change for 14 years. Only the development of the self-confrontation technique (described in Chapter 24) had any effect on him. He has now begun to change and to develop a more forgiving and positive self-image, although prognosis remains guarded.

THE UNREALISTIC SMALL PENIS COMPLEX

The majority of sex offenders I have seen in therapy will, at one time or another, "confess" that one of their unchangeable and most serious problems is that they have a small penis. When this occurs, should the therapist ask how big a normal penis should be the repetitive compulsive sex offender invariably will either not know or give some outrageous measurement that he has either heard from peers or has seen in some pornographic context (either pornographic books or videotapes).

Secondly, when asked in what context he has compared himself to other males of his age group, the repetitive compulsive sex offender invariably will state: in a shower, locker room, nude swimming situation, group physical line, etc. In these situations, the comparison is made to *flaccid* penises and, as the reader may be aware, this comparison is invalid due to the difference in retractability of the male genital organ. Penis size also depends a great deal on genetic background, race, etc. What the offender is unaware of, due to lack of adequate sex education, is that smaller flaccid penises tend to erect to a greater extent than larger flaccid penises do. Masters and Johnson [1982, p. 45] state:

> . . . men with a penis that is smaller when flaccid (non-erect) usually have a larger percentage volume increase during erection than men who have a larger flaccid penis.

Here again the sex offender has compared himself *upward* (see Chapter 2 and Ronny in Chapter 3) and through selective perception has ignored the other males in any of the comparison groups with either equal or smaller flaccid penises than his.

More important than his conclusion that he has a small penis is the value or importance that he attaches to it. In his distorted value system (see Chapter 18) a small penis makes him less of a man; unable to satisfy either a woman or a man; a failure (from birth); or justifies his deviant behavior.

If he is a pedophile or hebophile, he rationalizes that he will become involved with males of similar penis size, i.e., children or young adolescents. If he is a sexually assaultive person, then his use of force will prevent the woman or man from making comparisons or judgments about his organ size (especially at night or in the dark).

Lack of parental communication and lack of adequate sex education are both involved in the *misinformation* and *street or locker room knowledge* that the sex offender brings to therapy. Thus the importance of sex education programs in the overall treatment of this individual becomes especially obvious, especially in a group setting, since it was at a peer stage that the damage was done and it should be at a peer stage that the damage is corrected. Many self-help type sex education books are available today that will dispel sex misinformation while replacing it with the accurate and important facts he needs and wants to know.

Penis size, while a preadolescent/adolescent comparison behavior, is not the only sex education area where these individuals are misinformed and need to be reeducated. (See Chapter 24). However, it remains a prevalent and extremely important problem to sex offenders as a group. Another example will clarify the crucial role of penis size:

Bobby (introduced in Chapter 4) was in treatment for at least one, but possibly more rapes of adult women. There was no excessive force or brutality involved nor any sadistic injuries, but he did complete the rape and definitely traumatized the victim. An interesting element of his rapes was his insistence that the victim keep her eyes closed before he undressed and until he told her to open them after he redressed. He was not concerned about his identity as the detectives investigating the rape suspected or surmised. He simply did not want the victim to see his penis. Other rapists with the same problem and concern, accomplish the same end by raping in the dark, insisting that no lights be turned on or by blindfolding the woman. Again, the unknowing believe that this is only to protect the rapist's identity.

After many months in establishing trust and rapport in therapy, Bobby asked for an individual therapy (I.T.) session. As with other cases we discussed, it was time to reveal his big secret, which turned out to be his shame and embarrassment at having a small penis. When asked what a small penis is, he was unable to answer except to say that in his comparisons to his teammates in the gym locker room and in the showers, he didn't match up to any of them in size. These comparisons were made while he was in a flaccid state (the major error in this type of comparison by both teens and adults). I suggested that Bobby enroll in the next sex education course which was just about to begin a new semester and he did.

In teaching sex education with sex offenders, special emphasis must be placed on areas that especially concern this group more than others. These include: penis size, manhood values, responsibility for arousal and sexual behaviors, responsibility for pregnancy and sexually transmitted diseases (S.T.D.'s), the origin of their sexual values and how to change them, sexual preference versus sexual identity, etc.

After the second session, Bobby returned to my office, told me that he had listened to the range of normal penile dimensions and said that "his six inches was normal and okay with him."From that day on, his whole attitude changed and he became more assertive, competitive in sports (especially weight lifting) and his overall demeanor indicated a happier and more normal adjustment. Had this been done in grammar school or junior high school, the possibility exists that the rapes may have been averted. Creating an atmosphere where children and teenagers can talk about anything to parents or other adults they trust and respect is paramount in the prevention of sexual assault and abuse.

Pedophiles handle the small penis complex through distorted perception and delusional thinking. Even when they believe they have a small penis (and a large percentage of them do), they rationalize, quite accurately, that it will look larger to a small child by comparison. It is not too farfetched to believe that a percentage of them chose children as their victims from this type of thinking and motivation. An example will clarify:

☐ HOWIE *(whose case is discussed in Chapters 2 and 7) believed that he had not only a small penis but an abnormally small erection. This became a motivating force in his never allowing his victims to see him naked, except when they went skinny dipping and even then he remained in the water most of the time. When he was photographing them with erections or masturbating, he again was fully clothed and admired and envied their penises and wished "his was as beautiful and large as theirs."*

When, after several years of therapy, Howie had his first sexual experiences with other men, nothing they did could get him erect, although alone he had no such problem. In writing therapy, which was the only modality where he felt sufficiently comfortable to expose his feelings, thoughts and fantasies, he attributed his psychogenic impotence (his diagnosis) with other males to his fear of ridicule and laughter at his small erection capability. This fear and impotence remain to this day and there is no way to know whether his fears are real or imagined.

Finally, there is FRANK *(introduced in Chapter 2), who was told he had a small penis and would never be a real man, first by the babysitter who molested him, then by his sister during his first attempted heterosexual experience with her. During his rapes, he also never permitted his victims to look at his penis but did make them tell him what a great job he had done and how great a man he was.*

The *small penis complex*, when it originates early in childhood, leaves a definite *imprint* that lasts throughout life until resolved in therapy. This area is often overlooked by counselors and therapists who may be *uncomfortable* dealing with sexual issues. Without resolution of this problem, the rest of the therapy efforts are often wasted and the danger of recurrence of the deviate behavior or sexual dysfunction continues to exist.

DISTORTED SEXUAL VALUES

One of the most common traits or characteristics of the repetitive compulsive sex offender is his long-term value belief that *sex equals love.* This is the most frequently seen and most destructive of all the distorted values found in sex offenders.

In both pedophilia and hebophilia, the most often used rationalization by the offender to the victim when asked a "why" question about the sexual behavior is some reply containing the word love:

- I'm showing you *love.*

- We're making *love.*

- This is how two people show each other *love.*

- I want you to feel good because I *love* you.

The importance of uncovering this distorted, confusing and all-justifying value lies in the fact that what he has done, i.e., the sex crime or perversion, is therefore all right since he was *only showing his victim love,* not trying to harm him/her. This is especially true where the pedophiles and hebophiles are concerned, although I have heard it quite often from other sex offenders as well.

In their distorted perceptions and their overwhelming need to justify and/or rationalize their behavior (which they intuitively know is wrong), the belief that they love their victims is essential to alleviate the tremendous amount of guilt that they feel afterwards (assuming they are not sociopathic). This word, *love,* is used over and over in their contacts with their victims. It becomes imprinted in the victim's mind, as well, since the victim, after returning for the second, third and more contacts, is also experiencing guilt and needs his or her own rationalization to assuage the guilt. Thus the *merry-go-round* begins and, if not corrected through therapy, will be used in later years by the victim when he becomes the offender.

In a great many other sex offender case histories, a common thread in the offender's own molestation is the phrase "I'm showing or proving that I love you" in response to the child's question as to what the adult is doing to them. Especially when the child is lacking in all sexual knowledge and their molestation is their first encounter with genital sex, the *imprint* occurs immediately and lasts for life unless corrected in therapy.

☐ JIMMY *(an incestuous pedophile) was molested by his father from age nine to age 16 when he, in turn, began molesting his brother and sister as well as several younger children he babysat for. The first night, Daddy woke Jimmy sometime after midnight and took him into the spare bedroom. He undressed Jimmy and then himself (Jimmy, frightened, believed he was about to be beaten). He then began fondling Jimmy's genitals and ordering him to do the same to him. When Jimmy asked what was happening his father told him he was teaching him how to become a man and how to "make love" to a woman. He promised him that when he was good at sex, he would let him have sex with a real woman. Jimmy, having peeped at his parents having sex, was excited by the thought of "making love" like they did so he cooperated.*

When, after years of sex with his father and then with his younger sister (for "practice" under the father's direction), the promised sex with a real woman never occurred, Jimmy, feeling angry and betrayed, used any child he could manipulate and control, including two young boys he babysat for. Ironically, when his father was finally arrested for molesting his children, Jimmy, was arrested a few months later for molesting his siblings and was sent to the same institution that his father was sentenced to.

Their first session in therapy, together, was quite dramatic and extremely painful for both.

Jimmy, while molesting his younger siblings (both brothers and sisters) insisted that not only did they enjoy the sexual activities but it was the "best way I knew to show them that I loved them!"

As will be discussed in Chapter 18, the *source* of this value must be found before any change can be effected. Thus, let us consider how repetitive compulsive sex offenders learn values like this one.

In those sex offenders who themselves were molested the answer is obvious: They learned it from their molester who used it to justify his/her behavior toward the child and now they are using it in exactly the same way. This is the easiest to understand.

However, there is an even more insidious way is which this value becomes ingrained in young people today. Only in the United

States is the euphemism *"making love"* used to describe the act of sexual relations between two people. We still appear to be so sexually neurotic and puritanical, that to use any other phrase of a more direct nature to describe sex is either forbidden, too embarrassing or guilt-provoking to consider.

Imagine the effect on a young child, ERNIE, who accidentally (or otherwise) catches his parents in the violent throes of intercourse with accompanying audible dramatics and asks what they are doing only to be told "We're making love!" Now imagine some few days later when mother comes into his bedroom to find Ernie and his sister naked in bed "making love," and his mother's violent reaction. This actually happened to Ernie and his sister Laura. Mother began hitting Ernie with anything she could get hold of, all the while castigating him with epithets such as "disgusting, pervert, sickee," etc., and menacing him with threats of impending doom when his father came home. Ernie's father was even more violent and destructive in his reaction, literally beating Ernie into semi- consciousness and threatening to have him put in prison (a seven year old) all for "making love" as he had witnessed his mother and father doing. Needless to say, Ernie never forgot the incident and his attitudes and values toward sex were colored for life. Ernie, became a violent rapist and is in prison today.

DEVIANT AROUSAL PATTERNS

Still another unique trait or characteristic of the repetitive compulsive sex offender is the obsessive compulsive nature of his *deviant arousal patterns* for masturbatory or other sexual excitability needs. When the compulsion is active, the sex offender is unable to get aroused to a normal sexual stimulus or fantasy regardless of how hard he tries. If he does get erect, and a percentage do to anything that contains nudity or sexual suggestion, he is unable to reach orgasm unless he changes the fantasy to include his own subjective deviant stimulus pattern. For example:

> When Kevin watched his first sexually explicit film of a heterosexual couple in both foreplay and eventual intercourse (his choice of film), no matter how hard he tried to masturbate to orgasm nothing worked until in his own mind he altered

the content of the film to include force, submission and both fear and disgust on the part of the female. He then had an almost immediate orgasm and relief.

Jimmy, likewise, while watching a sexually explicit film of two adult homosexuals in foreplay, fellatio and eventual mutual anal sex (his choice of film), masturbated for over an hour. It only made him sore and he was no closer to a climax then he was during the first five minutes. He then switched the fantasy, in his own mind, making the younger looking of the two males a 13- or 14-year-old teenager, and immediately reached an orgasm.

There is a persistently seen resistance to *giving up the old stimuli subject* in both the pedophile/hebophile group and in the sexually assaultive person (S.A.P.) group, as well. They appear to prefer the security of their old and deviant fantasies to the risk involved in making changes. Their insecurity regarding new situations surfaces persistently, especially when change is the goal.

Attempting to *force change* through threat, success motivation techniques or through classical behavior modification techniques, in my experience, simply does not work. All that it accomplishes is confirmation of the offender's failure system and results in frustration and loss of confidence in treatment. The *Clockwork Orange* syndrome has been seen in hundreds of cases where either noxious odors, mild electric shock, or other aversive behavior modification techniques had previously been tried. [*Note* 1] The additional danger here is that the confidence of the offender in treatment itself may be shaken and the new therapist then has an additional resistance barrier to overcome before any meaningful therapy can begin.

As stated many times before, there are opposing views to mine, and the reader is once again referred to Dr. Pallone's coverage of alternate treatment techniques and their successes for other therapists (Pallone, 1990, Chapter 5). As will be discussed in Chapter 14, I have found from my own experience that a specific form of *masturbatory reconditioning* appears to be the best method of dealing with this problem when used in conjunction with the *value change* techniques discussed in Chapter 18.

A major caveat, in dealing with masturbatory homework assignments, is that they deal with *self-report*, the least reliable source of accurate information, especially where the sex offender is concerned. In the aftercare treatment I have conducted with paroled and maxed-out sex offenders for nearly 30 years, there has never been a single individual who has not admitted to me at some time in his aftercare treatment that he had lied during inpatient therapy, either directly or by omission. This occurs most often when the return of a deviant fantasy had occurred, especially if he was somewhere in the release process. The most commonly used justification is that he will handle it when he is released and that, if he admitted it at the time it occurred, he would be punished by being removed from the release process and delayed another year or more. It is only when the problem begins recurring in the community where real victims, not fantasy ones are available, that he panics and decides to admit it in an aftercare session.

The possibility that the offender has lied during therapy must be foremost as a consideration in evaluating the sex offender for possible release from incarceration or termination from treatment in private practice. A rule of thumb I have used for many years is to *believe nothing that the sex offender says unless it can be demonstrated behaviorally.* Where masturbatory reconditioning is concerned, this cannot always be applied and the therapist's decision must remain a judgment call, based on his experience and his therapy knowledge of the client.

NOTE

1 *A Clockwork Orange* is a novel by Anthony Burgess, published in 1963, which became a powerful film under the direction of Stanley Kubrick. The work is the psychological history of Alex, a delinquent 15-year-old in London at some unspecified future date, who has been conditioned to behave violently whenever he hears the strains of Beethoven's Ninth Symphony. Much of the dramatic conflict concerns the application of "Ludovici's Technique," a variant of aversive counter-conditioning — which becomes a matter of public controversy between members of opposing political parties. For an analysis both of the public policy and the clinical issues, see Pallone (1986, pp. 41-46; 1990, pp. 95-97).

8

Other Characteristic Deficits

DEFECTIVE GOAL-SETTING PATTERNS

As an extremist (typically), the sex offender avoids the middle-of-the-road norms and sets his goals either too high or too short ensuring failure on a persistent and repetitive level. This pattern appears to have been learned in early childhood from perfectionistic and well-meaning parents.

Report cards were particularly traumatic when school began and, in my experience at PTA meetings, parents continue making the same errors.

Remember the example in Chapter 2 of Billy and the seven-A and one-C report card? His parents' immediate reaction was "What's that C doing there?" The average child would extricate himself (or herself) from the situation easily by saying something to this effect: "Dad, that teacher wouldn't give her own son an A; for her a C is almost a miracle! How about a dollar for each A?" The sex offender, however, immediately feels guilt, shame and fear and becomes apologetic, promising that he will improve by the next report card.

Well-meaning parents *focus* their child's perception on the *negative,* and when this occurs, each time the child is in a situation that can be rated or compared to a norm, he may develop a permanent *negative self- perception* or focus. This becomes most damaging and dangerous if it continues into adolescence where comparison to peers is a primary activity. Constantly coming up below or inferior to his peer-group contributes to the inadequacy and low self-esteem mentioned earlier (see Chapters 2 and 3).

In addition, motivation is negatively affected as well and eventually (usually sooner than later) he may give up trying, since the pain of failure is too great. Thus, he will remain below potential in school, sports, social situations, etc. Either anger (for the sexually assaultive person) or a nostalgic return to an earlier, happier time (for the pedophiles and hebophiles) then dominates his fantasy life and, *if sexual trauma exists,* either sexual assault or pedophilia/hebophilia can result.

Allowing the child the opportunity to react to his performance, whether on a report card, in a competition or whatever, will give the parent an immediate clue that this process of *defective goal-setting* has begun. Then the opportunity exists to take corrective measures before the pattern becomes permanently ingrained. The longer the pattern has been there, the longer it will take to correct and, in some cases, while the perfectionism can be diminished or controlled, it appears that it cannot be totally erased.

EASILY DISCOURAGED — QUITS

Becoming easily-discouraged and quitting is a major barrier to change, and frustrates most efforts to help the offender to alter his past and present poor functioning. Most sex offenders have lived a life characterized by *failure.* These failures were either real failures or normal first time behaviors that others, primarily demanding, perfectionistic parents, characterized as failures. As we saw with Billy and his report card in Chapter 2, parents, whether well-meaning or simply sadistic, can set patterns of negative reference and focus for the child that may last for his whole life. This especially applies to weak, passive and inadequate personalities like the sex offender. When the therapist meets one of these clients as an adult with as many as 20 years of perceived failures and feelings of never quite being equal to his peers in anything, the problem is extremely difficult and complex. As with all of the other traits/characteristics of the sex offender, where the overall basic inadequacy results in less than normal functioning, so in this area also.

From the first meeting with this type of client, the focus must be on positives and the ambiance of the therapy-milieu must be totally positive, *while remaining realistic.* This is a difficult task at best, that requires a great deal of training and experience. Motivating the sex offender to *take risks* at attempting anything is a difficult, also at times impossible, task, whether it be to take the floor in his group, to expose a secret, to join an athletic team, to return to school to learn to read or write, to get his general equivalency diploma (G.E.D.) or take his first college course. He automatically sees *failure*, his greatest fear, as the outcome, regardless of his efforts or how hard he tries. He can readily quote his track record to prove his assumption.

Attempting to change this pattern without first getting him to understand its origin is frustrating and bodes failure on the part of the therapist. Analysis of his attempt patterns is essential and often uncovers the basic problem pattern. Usually one or both of the following goal-setting problems emerges.

1. Setting Goals Too High

In his need to deny/forget/change his perceived gross imperfections, the sex offender often tries to become perfect. *Perfectionism* thus becomes a major problem to expose and to deal with. Where goal-setting is concerned, the offender will set a goal to go from a C or D to an A rather than a C+; from striking out in a baseball game to hitting a home run, rather than simply not striking out or possibly getting a single; from never having spoken in group to taking the floor for the whole session and making it the best floor the group has witnessed; and he becomes involved in a constant *besting* process where peers are concerned. In reality, he does not for one moment believe he can accomplish any of these goals, nor has he taken the time or concern to evaluate his potential in each of the areas involved. Again he has *set himself up to fail* and thus returns to feeling sorry for himself and denigrating his abilities. It also becomes a prime reason not to ever try again, an excellent resistance factor for therapy. An example will clarify:

☐ FRED, *a pedophile/hebophile who prefers boys ages 11 to 14 as sex partners, applies for a job in the unit's computer center. During an interview with the supervisor he lists several computer languages as his forte and insists that he needs no training and wants to help in any way he can. The supervisor is quite impressed and asks if Fred thinks he can handle the construction of a totally new program in a fairly complex computer language. Fred immediately and enthusiastically volunteers for the task and says that he will have it completed in a month (the supervisor anticipated at least three to six months for completion). Fred begins the next day and, at the end of a week, presents a typed outline of how he perceives the project. Once again the supervisor is quite impressed, although by now he has received word from other programmers in the computer center that Fred is all talk and no action and that they do not believe that he is capable of completing the project, since he appears completely unfamiliar with the terminology of the language required (Pascal). Three more weeks go by and each time the supervisor has contact with Fred, Fred tells him that everything is going well and that he will meet his time-frame.*

As the supervisor has suspected, since a consultation with Fred's primary therapist, the deadline is not met and what work has been done on the program is useless. When questioned in the presence of his therapist, Fred tells the supervisor that he wanted so badly to succeed and please the supervisor and the treatment unit that he convinced himself that he would be able to quickly learn the language, even though he had had no prior experience with Pascal (an impossible task).

In therapy, Fred's group brought the subject of this failure up and eventually got Fred to confess that this was a pattern of his since grammar school and had cost him both friends and employment as well as punishment at home. In relating his story, Fred stated "I guess my father was right. I am a failure like he said I was, no matter how hard I try!"

Fred was unable to see his part in setting himself up to fail. Once he did, Fred began to tell the truth about his skills and abilities, and he set goals that were lower than his appraisal of his abilities. Thus he began to succeed.

The therapist must always be alert to this self-defeating pattern with the sex offender, not only in employment or educational abilities but also in relationships, social skills, athletics and every other facet of his life. If the pattern of failure is not aborted as quickly as possible, new failures will confirm his feelings of being worthless and will prevent the necessary new risk-taking behaviors that successful treatment will require.

2. Setting Goals Too Low (Short)

In his quest for success (often confused with perfection), the sex offender sets all-encompassing goals. For example, if he is going to learn to read, the goal will be to be able to read by the end of the first week; if weight loss is the goal, it will be 50 pounds in one week; if smoking is the problem, the goal is to quit the next day; if social relationships are the problem area, the goal is to meet and acquire many new friends the same day or by the end of that week. His unrealistic, black-and-white thought processes continue from childhood and failure is most often the result. Thus, through a *self-fulfilling prophesy* he sets himself up to fail and then can use each of these failures as an excuse to never try again, since the pain of failure is too great.

This problem of setting himself up to fail will occur in almost all aspects of his life including his therapy. Persistent failure becomes a way of life and a good alibi for feeling sorry for himself and doing something stupid or self-destructive as a kind of self-punishment. An example will clarify:

☐ MARK, *whom we met in several preceding chapters, was practically a non-reader and non-speller. This condition bothered him a great deal and produced shame, embarrassment and avoidance of any situation that required either task. Since it badly affected his self-image and self-esteem, the therapist tried to encourage him to attend school during the day, for which he would be paid. The treatment unit had several excellent teachers, trained specifically in remedial work. One female teacher,* MISS LAURA, *took a special interest in Mark. Together with the therapist, she was able to get him to sign up for classes at least six times in a three-year period. Mark would start each course all motivated and excited, but the first time he did not perform up to his demanding, perfectionistic expectations, he would quit. Regardless of the reality of his progress (which was quite normal for this particular class of non-reader, non-speller), he perceived failure. When his quitting was discussed both in individual therapy and in his group, he admitted that he knew he was going to fail even before classes ever began and, regardless of what his peers in the same class offered as positive or comparative feedback, nothing changed his mind.*

Nothing worked until his self-image and self-esteem began to change through *self-confrontation therapy* (see Chapter 21). Once these changes began, Mark returned to school and became one of the best and most successful students in the group. Within a year, he was reading and spelling at least six grade levels above where he began and, as a result, was able to get a highly technical job in the Video-Studio-Complex where reading maintenance manuals and submitting written reports and purchase orders was a primary task.

IDENTITY CONFUSION

In the last seven chapters, we discussed the individual traits and characteristics of the sex offender. *Identity Confusion* summarizes the total of all the other traits and becomes the overall identifier and main treatment consideration. This final trait/characteristic of the sex offender is the important and often unrecognized fact that: *he does not know who he is.*

If you give him a blank sheet of paper with the title *"Who Am I?"*, the response will contain a list of demographics but nothing about the persona of the individual. Name, age, sex, nationality, occupation, educational level, prior work experience, marital status, prior criminal history and possibly parental history will all appear, but there is no response to the real intent of the question. This is not resistance or evasion, as in other questioning, but a true lack of pertinent knowledge.

For the majority (if not the entirety) of his life, the sex offender has been what he perceived other people wanted him to be or, at best, a poor imitation of a peer or adult he admired and wanted to be like. If it worked and got him the attention, acceptance or other responses he wanted and desperately needed, he would assume the personality traits of anyone he had seen who had obtained satisfaction of such needs: a brother or sister, a friend in his neighborhood or a fellow student in school. This is one of the main reasons he can be so easily taken advantage of and/or abused without resistance.

An example from one of our already mentioned offenders will clarify the concept.

Kevin, as you will recall, came from a family with both parents, two brothers and three sisters. He perceived that the five other children had the acceptance and love from his parents that Kevin so desperately wanted and needed. He first tried to imitate his older brother who, when brought home by the police for some minor infraction, received attention, forgiveness and love from both parents. Kevin tried flashing, but instead of receiving love and acceptance, he was punished and rejected. Confused, he next tried to imitate his sisters, going so far as to cross-dress, and again was rejected and punished.

Later, in school, when he tried to imitate the more popular boys he again was rejected and ousted from the group he wanted acceptance from most. No matter what he tried it did not work and by young adulthood he was totally confused about his own identity. He developed a chameleon- like personality, imitating anyone and everyone he felt was popular or accepted. Anger continued to ferment during all of these episodes and became directed toward females, whom he perceived as most rejecting. As early as 11 years of age, he began fantasizing rape, and attempted his first rape during a flashing encounter when the girl laughed at his penis — an episode he may have perceived as her laughing at him.

A major treatment issue became, and still is, one of identity. More on Kevin later.

9

Treatment Issues: Overview

SOME PRINCIPLES OF CLINICAL INTERVIEWING

It goes without saying that, in order to expect to be effective in the treatment of sex offenders, the prospective "treater" must have mastered the clinical skills necessary for practice in one of the mental health professions of psychology, social work, psychiatry, or counseling. Even so, typical training programs for these professions rarely provide a sufficient base in specialized knowledge and clinical technique to permit the neophyte practitioner to plunge headlong into the task of treating sex offenders. Indeed, before we consider treatment principles and specific techniques particularly applicable to the treatment of these offenders, it is important to *know what we don't know*. Among the issues relevant to clinical interviewing in counseling or therapy with sex offenders are such concerns as these:

- Personal traits and characteristics that are essential for the counselor or therapist to possess if he or she is to work successfully with sex offenders.
- Treatment or therapy orientation/modalities that produce positive results with this population.
- Personality traits and defense mechanisms in both offenders and victims that facilitate or impede both disclosure and effective participation in treatment.

● CARDINAL PRINCIPLES IN CLINICAL INTERVIEWING

☐ *1. Readiness*
☐ *2. All the Nitty-Gritty Details/Facts*
☐ *3. Listening*
☐ *4. The Less Said by the Therapist, the Better*
☐ *5. Hope*
☐ *6. Body-Language*
☐ *7. Emotional Reactions*
☐ *8. Sensitivity to Lies or Manipulations*
☐ *9. Assume Nothing!*

- Specific barriers to revealing one's personal sexual molestation as a child.
- Means of assessing the reality or illusory character of purported changes in the offender.
- The function of *ritual* and *imprinting* in the pathology of the offender.
- Prognosis for effective treatment among the major offender groups: pedophiles, hebophiles, incestuous fathers, sexually assaultive persons.
- Distinguishing characteristics that boldly identify the personality of the true incestuous father.
- Needs unresolved in childhood that interfere with the relationship between the offender and his therapist, regardless of the sex of the therapist.

These nine cardinal principles, which cover the consistent problem areas I have encountered in supervising therapists new to this field, should be dealt with in some detail.

Readiness

Readiness on the part of the client and the therapist is a must prior to any interviewing attempt. In our experience, the client will let the therapist know when he/she is ready to get into the deeper or more serious issues, either by directly stating so or by leading statements and body-language, indicating that the client wants the therapist to ask questions or introduce more serious topics. Once this readiness is observed, the therapist needs to be ready for very heavy and emotional sessions.

Before any serious or factual discussion can take place, the *issue of confidentiality* must be thoroughly addressed. In the state where I practice, child abuse of any type must be reported, while all other sex offenses remain confidential unless the information poses a clear and imminent danger to the community. This law or any other legal factors or implications that could affect therapy must be explained to the client. The client must then be allowed to ask questions regarding these issues and must be given time to consider all of the ramifications before proceeding any further. My own preference is to cover this issue in the first session, before any serious material is discussed or accidentally related. The client then has at least a week to consider and to make a realistic decision.

Where very young children are concerned (my youngest was five years old) this issue must be discussed with the primary parent (the one bringing the child to the therapist and most involved in his/her care).

All the Nitty-Gritty Details

It is necessary to obtain *all the nitty-gritty details* of the client's past history the first time that the client is willing to talk about it. I strongly recommend that the therapist not allow generalities or vague and suggestive statements to substitute for the truth, or else the same areas will have to be gone over again and again to get the total picture.

It is quite common for children, adolescents and even adults to try to get away with telling as little as possible about their true problems, since telling the therapist all the terrible and traumatic details of their past and present problems means they must hear it again themselves and therefore relive it, to some degree.

Often, the client's operning statements resembles these:

- *"I had sex with him/her."*
- *"We did dirty or bad things."*
- *"I touched him/her."*
- *"We, you know, did it."*

Through encouragement and support, the therapist must elicit the rest of the material (the nitty-gritty details) in a direct but reassuring manner.

It is not uncommon, in an embarrassing, degrading or severely painful trauma, for the offender to reveal only the minimum that he/she feels is necessary. This is especially true in *rape* cases. Quite often the offender will leave out *the words he used, acts that are repulsive or disgusting,* or *the fact that she/he reached orgasm.* To accept minimum details can be misleading and prolong the therapy as well as delay any significant recovery.

An example, where this *almost* occurred may help to clarify:

☐ BOBBY, *(whose case is discussed in Chapters 4, 6 and 7) openly discussed the rape for which he was convicted with his first primary therapist. The therapist probed no further and within his first year of therapy wanted to refer Bobby for possible release from the program. When his therapist became ill and left the treatment facility, I inherited the case (at the therapist's request) and was willing to proceed with the release process after I had had a chance for an intensive interview. From the first 15 minutes or so something bothered me about Bobby's presentation. It was too pat and sounded very well-rehearsed. I informed him that I needed more time to get to know him before proceeding and also told him quite directly that I felt he was hiding something.*

Several weeks later, after Bobby had attended and participated in several of my groups, he requested an individual session. The first thing he mentioned was that his former therapy had not been as intense or as deep and that he felt there were issues that he needed to "confess." What amazed me was that his former therapist had never asked him about other rapes or sexual assaults for which he was never apprehended. This was the critical area. Bobby related the following: "... Sure there were other rapes, mostly all the same type and pattern except this one case." (At this point he appeared visibly frightened and tears began streaming down his cheeks.)

"This one lady was different from all of the rest. She laughed at me and said I was too small to rape anyone. I punched her as hard as I could and then ripped her pants and underwear off, saying 'I'll show you who's too small!' When I took my shorts off, she laughed crazily while pointing to my penis and said 'If that's all you've got, it'll get lost inside of me!' At that point, something happened and I went crazy. There was an old, broken baseball bat in the bushes where I had taken her and I picked it up and kept hitting her in the face and head with it until I couldn't hit anymore and until she was quiet. — Then I panicked and ran. I never saw anything in the papers about her but I think that she was dead."

Bobby had been treated for a year without ever mentioning this rape *because he was never asked about other rapes nor motivated to get all of the problems out and dealt with.* He had been terrified that someone would find out and that he would be tried for murder, so he never volunteered anything.

Now the total picture of the case changed. Not only was he an angry and dangerous rapist, but a potential murderer (the ultimate rape) as well. Were he released without this critical information uncovered, he would have raped again and possibly killed again. In following sessions, he made similar predictions on his own to his group. The fact that his rage had reached points of being uncontrollable and deadly had never been discovered or treated. Also, and of more importance, his motivations and the etiology of his rape behavior now had to be expanded to include both his body and penis size and important *triggers* that needed to be thoroughly dealt with before any possible return to the community.

Prior to this "confession," everyone who had worked with Bobby believed that the only precipitating factors involved in his rape behavior were his father's outrageous rejection and physical abuse and his mother's impotence at helping him (See Chapter 4). His good looks, likable demeanor and the sympathy and empathy everyone felt about his terrible childhood, made it easy for him to *hide* the true extent of his pathology and rage.

In trying to explain this essential factor to both therapists and new clients, I have often used the metaphor of making an appointment with a physician to discuss an embarrassing problem. If the patient leaves out specific and graphic details, due to fear of judgment, punishment or rejection, the doctor may make a wrong diagnosis and then prescribe the wrong medication and treatment. The patient will then be worse off than if he/she never went to the physician in the first place. Even small children are able to understand the significance of the metaphor.

It is also important for the therapist to define his or her own role to the client and assure the client that the therapist will not be judgmental or punitive.

Listening

In supervising many new therapists over the years, one of my most frequent criticisms has been that they have never learned to *listen*. Lecturing, preaching, interrupting, rapid-fire questioning, taking notes during the session, answering telephones and other forms of distraction replace the art of listening to what the client needs, and often must tell the therapist.

Lack of the necessary patience to wait until the client is *ready* to speak or to continue often disrupts his/her concentration and train of thought or, even more frequently, gives the client an excuse to *forget* what they were relating in the first place. As stated in prior sections, the offender will use any excuse or alibi to get away from a sensitive, embarrassing or guilt-provoking area and, too often, the therapist provides the way out.

I have experienced pauses of as long as three to five minutes, a seeming lifetime of silence in a therapy session. Usually the wait is worth it, because the client is fighting with himself/herself about revealing something difficult, betraying a confidence or identifying an abuser. The *pause* often identifies the crucial areas and/or subjects for the therapist, if he/she is paying attention.

The Less Said by the Therapist, the Better

In order to accomplish good listening skills and yet keep the session moving, I suggest the use of a few, well-placed, *cue-words* which will be discussed more fully in Chapter 10 under the section on Confrontation:

- *Because?* — For statements/feelings without reasons.
- *And?* — There must be more to the thought/statement.
- *Pzzzzzzt!* — A polite I don't believe you.
- *Picture?* — I don't understand. Make me see it.
- *Tilt!* — You're off the subject. Get back to it.
- *Belly-Button!* — Used where behavioral changes are concerned. Means don't tell me you've changed, prove it to me by examples.

Where this skill is concerned, experience will always be the best teacher.

Hope

At the first opportunity, it is important for the therapist to communicate to the client that:

- While offenders are sick and have problems, this does not mean they are totally bad people; it means they are human beings with a problem.
- The future depends on working through all of the facts and feelings, especially any *anger/rage* reactions that may still be there from childhood trauma.
- While the full responsibility for the offense is the client's, he or she can be treated and eventually lead normal and happy lives. In other words, *there is help.*
- The past does not predict or determine the future, and *change is possible and can be permanent.*
- Offenders need a return to *reality* — not judgment, punishment, distortion, etc.
- Offenders need to identify and resolve *all guilt* for their past and present deviant behaviors in order to live normal and healthy lives in the future.

Body Language, Choice of Terms, Adjective, and Emotional Reactions

Once the therapist has mastered the skill of listening, learning to concentrate and pay attention to anything and everything the client says or does is paramount in importance. A change of position, change of facial expression, a sudden downward glance or avoidance of prior eye contact, all signal to the attentive therapist that a sensitive, painful or guilt-producing area may have been broached. Depending on the situation, the therapist may choose silence with some form of physical support, such as simply nodding his/her head or moving or leaning closer. The therapist may also choose some form of verbal support, from the simplest *"Uh huh"* to *"Take your time"* or *"Are you okay?"* or *"Do you want to continue?"* The therapist, at this point, must know the client and know what is most appropriate for the particular situation.

One important word of caution: under no circumstances should the therapist use the too-frequently stated *"I understand."* Where the offenders are concerned, unless the therapist himself/herself has been a sex offender or victim of sexual abuse, rapport can be lost with this one patronizing statement. Instead of seeming supportive, it will most likely produce anger in the offender and a loss of credibility for the therapist, thus damaging essential rapport.

I have observed this reaction on videotape countless times, when a new or inexperienced therapist under supervision makes this critical mistake and then cannot understand the client's reaction of anger and hostility. One such case comes to mind:

☐ *A young male psychologist, just out of graduate school with his Master's degree and freshly out of a clinical internship in a state mental hospital, was conducting his first interview with a 20-year-old male who was a pedophile and himself had been molested. Early in the first interview, the man stated: "It was terrible! Awful! The worse thing that ever happened to me! I feel dirty and contaminated!"*

Without the least hesitation or time to think the young psychologist replied: "I know, I know! I understand just how you feel." Immediately the client became enraged, stood up and yelled down at the stunned psychologist: "Oh, yeah!! When did you get fucked in the ass?"

The psychologist stammered something so quietly it was not picked up on the videotape and the man left the room, slamming the door. The therapist forgot the following important principle concerning survivors of sexual abuse.

Survivors Are Extremely Sensitive to Lies of Manipulations

A more appropriate response by the therapist would have been "It certainly must have been a terrible experience for you. I really don't know what you must have gone through but I'd like to, if you would share it with me." This example presents support, as well as a chance to gain trust with honesty and to encourage the client to continue and go into further detail in order to get the therapist to understand.

Where *choice of terms, adjectives and emotions* are concerned, the therapist will be most effective and miss the least amount of important material if the following principle is followed.

Assume Nothing!

In training new therapists, I always suggest that where any form of sexual deviation is concerned, regardless of the age of the client, the therapists act as if they had just arrived from another planet and need every word, phrase and term clearly defined and explained by the client. Using the therapist's own background knowledge or personal experiences can cause confusion and lose valuable material while it is fresh in the client's memory. This is especially true in the session where the facts of the abuse are first divulged.

A tragic example can best illustrate this all important point:

☐ TONY, *is now a young 23-year-old adult. When he was only slightly more than 15, he was sent to the old New Jersey State Diagnostic Center on a charge of juvenile delinquency involving impregnating his 14 year old sister,* JILL. *Since both Tony and his sister admitted the charges, the case seemed cut and dried and the only diagnostic or therapeutic work left was to decide on a course of action. The choices were to return Tony to his home under strict supervision, or to send him to a reformatory for punishment (since there was little treatment available in those days.)*

However, my gut reaction was that there was something amiss in this case. Tony just seemed wrong for this particular charge and there was definitely something unusual about the whole family. The social worker on the case was asked to do an in-depth workup on the family while I decided to do some brief therapy with Tony on an emergency basis. Following the principles outlined above, I asked Tony to make believe that I was from another planet and knew nothing about the reproductive behavior of humans. Smiling, he agreed and thought this would be an interesting game. I then instructed him to take me through the impregnation of his sister, step by step, leaving nothing to my imagination. The following story emerged.

Due to money problems, Tony and the other children were only allowed one bath per week. Since he was the oldest, he went first. To save money, he was not to drain the water but leave it for his sister to bathe in. Being a normal adolescent, he became stimulated washing his genitals and proceeded to masturbate and ejaculate. Jill then bathed, not knowing what Tony had done, and a month or more later announced that she was pregnant. When Tony was questioned by his parents he admitted to the masturbation in the bathtub, and they told him that that was how his sister became pregnant and that he was the father.

When I recovered from my shock at the story, I asked Tony about intercourse and he admitted that the whole family played the "fun games" on a regular basis: Tony with his mother, and his sister with her father. The younger children were allowed to watch and were taught to pleasure themselves with masturbation. When asked about babies, Tony stated that they were a gift of God. He did not connect pregnancy to the "fun games" in any way whatsoever. I then spoke to Jill, who was also at the center, and she readily admitted playing "fun games" with several of the boys on the football team at school. She also discussed her "fun games" with her father.

The social worker on the case was informed and reluctantly discussed the "fun games" with the parents who, surprisingly, readily admitted that this was their only pleasure since they couldn't afford T.V. or other entertainment, and that it was the best way to show their kids *that they loved them.* Needless to say the parents were evaluated and found to be of borderline intelligence, and socially isolated and retarded.

The real trauma in this case, resulted from the arrest, exposure, ridicule by peers and neighbors, and the deriding and callous attitude of the juvenile officers. Needless to say, the family had to be relocated. A total program of re- education and resocialization training was undertaken and both Tony and Jill were provided therapy. Jill had her baby and, due to the unusual circumstances, the parents were allowed to adopt the child as their own. Supervision was provided by the then Bureau of Children's Services.

Through psychological testing, Tony was found to be of above-average to superior intelligence and, with a great deal of tutoring, improved in his school work sufficiently to go to a community college.

Without *"assume nothing!"* as a guide and without following up on *gut reactions,* the true facts of this case would never have emerged; Tony and Jill would have ended up in reformatories and the rest of the young children would have continued to be sexually abused. It is important to state here that I have encountered hundreds of cases *where the surface facts in no way reflected the true facts of the case.*

TERMS

The client's choice of words can tell the therapist a great deal about how he/she feels about what happened, how much guilt exists and how judgmental the client is being about himself/herself. Also, the rapport, trust and confidence that the client has will be exposed in word choices as well as spontaneous emotional reactions. For example, for an adolescent boy or young adult male to use slang sex terms rather than precise anatomical ones may indicate greater trust and rapport with the therapist and may also increase credibility.

Adding an adjective to a term may clearly indicate the degree of guilt, anger or pain that the client is communicating. "It was dirty, filthy, disgusting and sickening" is far different than "It was terrible." Keeping track of these terms and adjectives enables the therapist to measure desensitization and progress over a period of time and indicates when the next level of therapy can begin.

Clients with very low self-esteem and who are resistant to seeing themselves in a better light, frequently use minimizing phrases, including:

- "Sort of."
- "A little bit."
- "Maybe."
- "No big deal."

and many others. These phrases are most frequently used in discussing some positive change or risk or new behavior that the client has accomplished. When asked if the particular behavior is positive, an affirmation is immediately minimized and the head goes down and the voice deepens and trails off.

Dennis (see Chapters 6, 12, 13 and 14) usually begins all sessions with a litany of failures, errors, mistakes and homework assignments he did not do because "I guess I didn't want to." When this negative confessing is complete, he will then add one or two occurrences that he felt could be seen as positive: "Well, I did call one of my friends and ask him to go to a concert with me. We really had a good time — *but the only reason he went with me is because he had a fight with his girlfriend and had nothing better to do.*"Or: "I went for a new job interview and they hired me. It's quite a promotion and really good for my future — *but I'll probably screw it up like I do everything else.*" In feedback, the therapist who pays close attention to these terms and listens to what the client is really trying to communicate can then use the same terms and inquire as to why they are always appended.

Reverse role-play also helps in these instances. I like to use one of the client's close friends, whom he really cares about, in the role-play. In its simplest terms, the technique involves repeating the same phrases —*as the friend*— and then asking the client how he would respond. The answers are usually right on target. The client now is in a "Catch 22" situation since if he tries to talk the friend out of the minimizing behavior, the therapist can ask why he doesn't do the same for himself. If he allows the minimizing by his friend, then he really doesn't care about the friend or want to make him feel better.

The focus of all these types of sessions has to be aimed at *reality* and *balance*. With very difficult and resistant clients, the technique I use is to *forbid* them to use a second negative judgment about themselves until there has been at least a one positive judgment. Thus, one negative, followed by one positive, followed by the second negative, followed by the second positive, etc. Eventually the concept of *balance* takes hold and they are able to relate a week's events in a more realistic manner.

GROUP VERSUS INDIVIDUAL TREATMENT

Of all of my major errors (and therefore learning experiences), *emphasizing and depending on individual therapy* was the most serious. The seductive and manipulative personality of the offender should be one of the most important of all therapeutic considerations. These individuals can perform well enough to win an academy award and thus the danger of the therapist being fooled, used or manipulated exists for whatever goal the sex offender chooses (especially freedom).

As a group, however, they become an ideal ruler to measure the change or lack of change of their fellow group members. While this is unusual in a correctional or institutional setting and would be considered *ratting* under normal circumstances, this confrontive exposure of their peer's behavior appears to serve several functions:

- It helps to assuage their intense guilts.
- They feel it will earn acceptance from the therapist.

- It prevents guilt from occurring should they allow a group member to deceive the therapist, be released and another victim results.

GROUP "MUSTS"

Direct But Don't Interfere.

While the therapist needs to remain in control and directive, new supervisees tend to take over the group and become lecturers or teachers. In fact, I have supervised some who could not run a group without a blackboard. While some instruction in group procedures may be necessary, once these initial sessions are over, the group should be allowed to run pretty much on its own with the following control functions performed by the therapist.

Keep the Focus of the Session or Topic.

Groups tend to lose focus quite easily and quite often. Also, the man-on-the-floor may deliberately change the subject when the going gets too emotional, painful or threatening to his image or security. The therapist's role, at this point, is to keep the group and the subject on course until some conclusion is reached or the subject can no longer continue.

Don't Take Sides or Become Judgmental

A serious group error that many therapists make is to become the protective parent on behalf of the client who is being confronted, facing anger from the group or appears totally alone in his views. This is especially true when a "seductive little defenseless boy" type offender is being picked on by the stronger bullies in the group. Helping him to grow up, face these negative reactions, and see that he will survive becomes an important therapeutic benefit when the therapist *stays out of these battles between individuals and the group.* If the therapist uses these times and situations to *observe,* he/she will learn a great deal, not only about the man-on-the-floor, but also about many of the other group members.

Becoming judgmental destroys the rapport and trust that the group and its individuals need in order to believe that the therapist's main motive is to help them. One instance of this type may permanently change the trust between the therapist and the group that is necessary for it to be functional and productive.

Never Give Answers, Ask Indirect Questions

The danger here should be obvious. Due to the strong defense mechanisms of the offender, the therapist will often see answers and insights long before the offender does. At times it is both difficult and frustrating not to *suggest* an answer or direction, but this must be avoided. If the therapist suggests an insight or answer that the client has been struggling with, the offender will usually accept it in order to please and agree with the parent- authority-figure, and the therapist will never know for sure whether the verbalized insight is truly the client's own. *It is more important for the client to find his own answers,* regardless of the amount of time this may take. Each offender, as we have previously stated, is a unique individual and, while the therapist may sincerely believe that he knows where the client is coming from and that he has heard the answer before, the possibility that this is a new and never-before-heard insight always exists.

Also, if a solution suggested by the therapist fails, the offender will place the blame (and rightfully so) on the therapist and refuse responsibility. Since making the offender accept responsibility is a major role of this therapy, the error is obvious. An example will clarify:

☐ *Early in my work with offenders, I met and treated* LUKE *another Vietnam veteran who was married and had a son that he adored. Luke was arrested for performing fellatio on pre-teen and teenage boys, whom he paid for the act in order to keep them from telling anyone. One of his pickups apparently was more innocent and naive than the others he had molested and went home and told his parents what had happened. Luke was arrested.*

Luke was quite a likable individual and all of his group and quite a few other therapists and staff at the treatment center knew him and felt positive towards him. In therapy, he was open, honest and a hard worker. He worked with the Vietnam veterans group as well. What was quite obvious was the amount of guilt that Luke was suffering from something besides his sexual offenses (guilt from his violent, sadistic sexual and killing behaviors in Vietnam). After a little over three years of therapy in which I felt Luke had made tremendous progress, I began preparing him for possible release. His family visited regularly and Luke and his wife seemed to be a loving couple with an adorable and quite bright son whom Luke adored.

Whenever Luke balked at the thoughts of release, I pressured him on behalf of his family and assured him that he could continue in an outpatient setting with little or no problem. Luke finally agreed and was released shortly after. He returned to his old job, where he was welcomed by his employer and fellow workers with open arms. He did not have to begin at the bottom all over again but instead was given a promotion. Everything looked wonderful! For a year or so, all appeared well and in outpatient, Luke reported no problems or recurrences of fantasies or impulses.

A week after his first year anniversary on parole, Luke was arrested, caught in the act with a 12 year old boy in his car.

In our first interview upon his return, I asked what happened and he angrily screamed at me: "I told you I wasn't ready but you kept insisting that I was! I trusted your judgment more than my own and look what happened to me and my family." It was later revealed that Luke's first recurrent act with a young boy occurred only a week or two after release. He "played the game" for his wife and child as well as the friends who had so much faith in him. The guilt from Vietnam had never been resolved.

From that day forward, I made it a practice to put *all responsibility for evaluation of therapy progress* on the individual. Now, even when a client says he/she feels that he/she is ready for promotion, I deny it and make him/her prove it. *"Show me, don't tell me!"* has become my stock phrase in such situations. In addition, should the client prove through behavior that he has made significant progress and is ready for promotion or termination (Prn Status), I then look for confirmation from others who have daily contact with him. Without these two proofs no promotion or change in program is given.

HOMOGENEITY OF GROUPS

One of the persistent areas of controversy in the treatment of the offender is that of *homogeneity of groups*. While we have already discussed the vast differences in the personalities of the different types of offenders (and will continue to do so in the following chapters) their *sameness* is far more important as a treatment issue. Another concern is the danger of their forming a mutual defense block against the therapist. Therefore mixing types of offenders in groups has been far more productive for us, and has kept the groups alive and interesting.

It is incredible to see the interaction of the different types of offenders and their *self-determined hierarchies.* Each feels that the other's choice of deviant behavior is far worse than his own (a minimizing mechanism), and cannot understand the other's choice of victim or deviant act. The most common hierarchies I have encountered are represented in the following statements:

- *Rapist:* "At least what I did was *normal* and with an adult woman, not kids like those perverts!"

- *Incestuous father:* "How could those deviates molest someone else's kid? That's disgusting! — I only used my own kid and I had that right, they didn't."

- *Hebophile:* "I can't understand those guys having sex with six and seven year olds. There's nothing there and they can't really do anything. It doesn't make sense!"

- *Pedophile:* "It wasn't sex. It was sex education and loving! What those others did was dirty and awful. I only showed my victims tenderness and how to feel good."

- *Flasher:* "I don't know why I'm even here! I never hurt anyone. All these other guys are criminals, I'm not. No one ever got hurt from seeing a guy's penis."

In a group setting, these perceptions of each other play an important confrontational role. In trying to understand each other's deviate behavior, questions abound. As a result, in a well functioning group, the therapist can almost sit back as an observer; the groups tend to run themselves.

On the other hand, when we tried a group of all pedophiles, the therapy was unsuccessful because they were so passive, frightened and unable to be confrontive, all that occurred was mutual support, exchange of experiences and sharing of new fantasies for their nightly masturbation. Little or no progress or change occurred and resistance became stronger rather than diminishing.

TYPICAL GROUP ERRORS SEEN IN SUPERVISION

In almost 30 years of supervising therapists with sex offenders and victims, I have witnessed the same errors again and again. Below is a list of the most common mistakes that I have observed:

- Beginning the group with an adversarial role on the part of the therapist.
- No empathy or observable interest on the part of the therapist.
- Threats by the therapist to the group or an individual in the group.
- Lack of education of the group into the concepts of group process or therapy rules/roles.
- Use of force by badgering the members of the group or one individual in the group.
- Too much interpretation on the part of the therapist.
- Ignoring readiness concepts and trying to force admissions/confessions too soon.
- Taking control too soon.
- Becoming too defensive.
- Playing the victim of the group when things do not go the therapist's way.
- Alienating the group by demands, too much control, forced topics or direction.
- Much too much talking or involvement on the therapist's part.

These observations will be discussed in greater depth as we progress in our discussion of the treatment of the sex offender.

10

The Four C's of Sex Offender Treatment

There are four principles or cautions that are readily identifiable as necessary mandates in sex offender treatment. These principles are summarized in tabular form in this chapter. Each of these elements will be considered in some detail with examples where applicable.

CONFRONTATION BY THE THERAPIST

Due to the passivity, dependency and seductiveness of the sex offender, there is a tendency on the part of therapists to be supportive, gentle and parental in their approach. In our experience, we have found that none of the supportive, passive therapies (including Rogerian, Psychoanalytic and other techniques of this type) worked for us. Naturally, there will be divergent views on this point. What we are discussing is our own personal experience with sex offenders.

One reason for our stance is that the offender's *denial* is so intense and the guilt so great that admitting the offense(s) is too traumatic and is avoided at all costs. As stated before, not all of our colleagues will agree with this stance and, for a contrary view, the reader is referred to Dr. Nathaniel Pallone's excellent coverage of

---

● THE FOUR C's OF SEX OFFENDER TREATMENT: CONFRONTATION, CAUTIONS, CONFIRMATION, CONSISTENCY

1. CONFRONTATION

☐ *a. Non-directive, passive type therapies usually fail.*

☐ *b. The therapists must be active, take control, confront.*

☐ *c. Value change is the most essential focus, followed by new self-image formation.*

☐ *d. Use of questions, not answers produces better results.*

2. CAUTIONS

☐ *a. Sex offenders are manipulative, seductive and con-artists.*

☐ *b. Rationalization, projection and denial dominate as the most frequently used defense mechanisms.*

☐ *c. Explosive reactions are possible — and unpredictable.*

3. CONFIRMATION

☐ *a. Believe nothing sex offenders say.*

☐ *b. Use group therapy to confirm changes and/or, new patterns.*

☐ *c. The therapist's comfort with sexuality.*

☐ *d. Relatives, staff and family are necessary partners to confirm facts, changes and new behaviors.*

4. CONTINUATION/CONSISTENCY

☐ *a. Aftercare treatment is essential.*

☐ *b. Emergency access to his former therapist is necessary.*

☐ *c. Consistent treatment is important.*

---

other sex offender treatment techniques in his *Rehabilitating Criminal Sexual Psychopaths* (1990).

In my experience, whether in individual or group settings, *confrontation* appears to be the only method that will reach the core of the sex offender's problems. Whatever the offender says, it must be doubted and he must always be made to back up or prove his statements. The offender either tends to use vague generalities and/or quickly picks up and uses psychological jargon as a means of mitigating or minimizing the impact of his statements. After confrontation, the vague statement "I molested my daughter" becomes: "I forced my daughter to fellate me and forcibly sodomized her."

When using confrontation it is important not to interrupt the thought processes of the client with long-winded statements and/or questions. Thus, we developed an easily learned and understood *cue phrase* system to prevent this interruption being used as a means of avoidance by the client.

Although already presented in Chapter 9, these cue phrases are important enough to repeat in this section as suggestions.

- *Picture* — You're being vague and I don't get a clear understanding of the situation.
- *Because* — I don't understand the motive or reasons for your actions/conclusions.
- *Pzzzzzzt* — I don't believe you or I don't buy that explanation, reason etc.
- *Show Me* — Don't just tell me the changes you've made, give me proof that I can verify.
- *And?* — Not enough. Whatever you're telling me is incomplete. Something is missing.
- *Tilt* — You're off the subject or track! Get back to what we were discussing.

The principle involved here is that *the less said by the therapist, the better.*

Nondirective, Passive Type Therapies Frequently Fail

The sex offender's defenses, especially denial, minimization, projection, avoidance and evasion, all demand a confrontational approach. In my experience, weeks, months and even years can be spent in frustrating therapeutic contact with these clients with no visible change or improvement when passive methods are used. (Here, again, refer to Pallone [1990] for divergent opinions on this topic.)

Often new therapists in the treatment of sex offenders, have been trained in these passive type treatment modalities and insist they will work. I always encourage them to give it a try, and within a short period of time (usually fewer than three months) they return and acknowledge that, *with this type of offender these methods do not work.* Then real training begins.

The Therapist Must Be Active, Take Control, Confront

Until a new group is well-trained and can function fairly independently, the therapist must direct, control and keep the group on track. Since *avoidance* of any painful topic of reexperience is part of the offender's makeup, he will try any tactic to change the subject, get off on a tangent and lead the group discussion away from the feared topic. The therapist must be alert and constantly keep the group focused on the topic of the man on the floor (the individual presenting his topic or problem to the group).

There is also a danger of the group *harming rather than helping* the man on the floor. Sex offenders become quite judgmental of each other, since they can feel better about themselves by finding someone more deviant or depraved than themselves. It is extremely important that the therapist allow sufficient time (usually ten minutes) at the end of each group meeting for:

- Recovery from an emotional session;
- A summary of what occurred in the session;
- Each group member to give his own feedback to the man on the floor.

During feedback the therapist should always be last. It is also important that the therapist's feedback show no favoritism or partiality (such as defending the man on the floor from the group) and that plans/goals for the next session be clearly delineated.

Focus on Value Change and Formation of a New Self-Image

All sex offenses are based on one or more seriously defective values, learned from early childhood and distorted to fit the deviant needs of the offender. Value formation and change are discussed in greater detail in Chapter 21. For this section, allow it to suffice that this is one of the most difficult, frustrating and long-term battles that the therapist will face.

Use Only Questions, Not Answers

A common error of the new therapist is giving the client cues and answers. For example:

- "That really must have been a frightening and awful experience!"
- "That really must have made you angry!"
- "You really must have hated him/her for that!"
- "You really must feel guilty about what you did to your daughter!"

instead of:

- "I've never had that happen to me. Can you help me to understand how it felt to you?"
- "When he/she did that, how did you feel?"
- "When it was over and you had time to think about it, what did you feel about the incident?"

It is important to remember that asking questions that don't give hints of the expected or desired answers is an art. Unfortunately, there is not enough emphasis put on this issue in the formal training of therapists. *Supervised practice* utilizing videotape (the ideal method) or audiotape, is the ideal way to learn. Tape playbacks, especially videotape, instantly expose errors in the words or facial and body language of the client. Sudden loss or gain of eye contact, a shift in sitting position, head down or suddenly up, tension from a relaxed state, etc., all instantly betray the reaction of the client to any statement by the therapist, either in individual therapy or in group. While audio taping is helpful, the *visible clues* are lost and the supervisor must rely on the accurate recall of the supervisee.

It should be mentioned that sex offenders are constantly *looking for answers* and want the therapist to provide them. They will try anything to accomplish this goal and, if they do, can then deny the answer at any future time and blame the failure on the therapist. Some typical questions that offenders want the therapist to answer include:

- "What should I do with my life?"
- "What changes should I make?"
- "What goals should I set?"

- "When do you want to see me again?"
- "Why do you think that I did it?"
- "What makes me do these things?"
- "Should I go to A.A. or N.A. or some other ancillary program?"
- "Should I tell my wife? parents? friends?"

Each of the above is a *trap*! Once the therapists answers the question, all future blame for the consequences of the choice becomes the therapist's and not the client's. If for example, the therapist suggests that the offender tell his wife of the offense and she then leaves and divorces him, the client may conclude that she left him not because he committed a sex offense but because he told her about it and that is the therapist's fault. The same follows for all of the other hundreds of questions that the sex offender will ask the therapist to answer during the course of treatment.

CAUTIONS

Sex Offenders Are Manipulative, Seductive, Con Artists

Most offenders I have met in either private practice or in an institutional setting were nice people. They are polite, gentlemanly, cooperative, well-behaved and very hard workers. They do everything they can to please and be accepted. It is quite common for them to make the therapist the positive parent that they never had and to try to create a personal relationship for themselves with the therapist.

In this dynamic there is also a means of *normalizing* themselves and feeling equal to the therapist. When this occurs the sex offenders distance themselves from their peers and see themselves more as part of the staff rather than part of the client population. Once this delusion is accomplished, their normal *denial mechanisms* take over and they no longer are the dirty, bad, evil perverts that were sent for treatment. Thus the therapist must constantly guard against this type of relationship developing.

Female therapists are at even greater risk since, if the offender can delude himself into believing that his therapist *wants* him as a boyfriend, he will misperceive even the most innocent kindness for love and soon become infatuated with the therapist. Usually she is the last to know that this is what he really feels and when it becomes known, (through love letters, touching, gifts, etc.) it is often too late to deny it since the offender will find a rationalization for the denial:

- "The authorities made her say that!"
- "She's worried about her job; but when I get out, then we'll be lovers."
- "She really loves me but has to be fair to the rest of the group."
- "She doesn't know she loves me but I'll convince her."

The dangers here are apparent and must be avoided even through transferring the client to another therapist's caseload.

Rationalization, Projection, and Denial Dominate as Defense Mechanisms

While sex offenders tend to overuse all of the defense mechanisms, the three defenses discussed here tend to dominate.

Rationalization, projection and denial exist from the first contact with the offender and contain the excuses, alibis and explanations for his behavior; why he could not have done it or why it happened.

The therapist needs to find a method of getting the offender to see and accept the reality of the situation. Because it will be painful for the offender to accept full responsibility for the act, the therapist must take his/her time to avoid making him face too much too soon. If the offender's initial experience with therapy is extremely painful and frightening, it is more than possible that he will quit therapy, if not physically then mentally by lack of concentration or involvement. It is more useful in the long run to allow the original defenses to exist and then, as rapport and confidence build, to slowly break through the defenses with specific questioning and a persistent return to the defended area. An example will clarify:

☐ JOEL, *a 29-year-old mechanic and part-time musician, was convicted of child molestation involving two children he was babysitting. From his first intake interview he was in total denial and insisted that he pled guilty rather than put the two children through the ordeal of testifying in court. He was one of the best adjusted individuals that the institution had. He was a gentleman, honest, kind, a hard worker, a good friend to many other sex offenders, and was generally liked by everyone. In group, while a consistent participant for others, when he took the floor, he discussed his alcohol and drug problems, his concerns for his family and especially an ailing father and other situational and adjustment problems — anything but his offense.*

If pressed to discuss the details of his charges, Joel strongly (almost angrily) stated that he was not a sex offender. He would then repeat his rationalization as to how he was convicted. After several years of therapy and watching other friends and group members "bare their souls" and improve both emotionally and psychologically, he took the floor in group and now changed his story. The second version became: "It might have happened. I was so drunk and so high on drugs that I really don't remember what happened that night. But, I'm still not a sex offender and I'm definitely not turned on by kids." Although both the group and the therapist did not believe this new version, he was encouraged to keep working in therapy and to try to remember what really happened that night in his apartment.

More than a year passed, and the third version emerged:

"I've begun to remember something about that night. I wanted to have a party and invited my friends over. This dizzy dame that I can get drugs from sometimes came along with one of my other friends, and the dumb bitch brought her two young kids with her. Eventually they went to sleep on the day bed. — After a few hours, we were all kinda high but the drugs were running low and she decided she would go get some more. She took the keys to my car and left, without even asking. Several hours later, everyone left and I was stuck with her damn kids. I sat near the day bed staring at them and then went over and sat on the bed. I was really horny from the drugs and maybe, I don't remember this part, touched the little girl but only through her clothes, not in her pants like the report says."

Revenge was now his rationalization and the blame was *projected* onto the mother of the victims. He was still in total denial that he could possibly have pedophilic tendencies or traits. This level remained unchanged for several more years. When asked why he would choose sexual contact as a way to hurt the mother of the children, he could not answer.

Shortly after this admission, Joel decided to max. While he continued to attend his group, no further therapy progress occurred. He is now back in the community and only time will tell if he will repeat.

Explosive Reactions Are Possible — and Unpredictable

The therapist should never become too complacent or comfortable when dealing with sex offenders and their problems. Most offenders have problems in the area of emotional expression and *"stuff"* their feelings in the present as they have done since they were children. As children they were never permitted this emotional expression and usually there is a great deal of suppressed anger that may erupt when the right buttons are pushed. Since the therapist is working in the dark where the past is concerned (only has what's in the record or what the client has shared), he/she can never know when an explosive reaction will occur. A personal example will illustrate:

☐ *During one of my groups with offenders,* RICHIE, *the man scheduled to have the floor, did not show up for group. Since he worked on the kitchen crew and had had problems getting off of work before, I made a phone call and had him sent to the main studio where we were videotaping his group. When he arrived he looked the same as always, and I asked why he had held the group up for over 15 minutes. He stared at me for a moment, took off his shoes (a safety rule in the studio), walked over to one of the video cameras (a $7,000 unit on a rolling tripod), calmly picked up the whole camera unit and attempted to kill me by bashing in my head. He missed me by about an inch and then, roaring, threw another camera through the one-way window between the studio and the control room.*

In about 30 seconds the entire group was up and jumped Richie. He simply threw them around the room as though they weighed nothing. In about a minute and a half, he threw up his hands, said "It's over!" and calmly sat on the floor and awaited the officer-help that had been summoned. Richie had never shown any anger outbursts in his many years of serving time and was always seen as a large but friendly "pussy cat" whose behavioral record was excellent. In checking his record there were no recorded incidents of violence, and even in his rape (the offense he was in prison for) he was nonviolent and, in fact, took the victim home after the incident (which led to his capture). In the many more years Richie would serve on his sentence, he never again showed any aggressive or violent behavior and I eventually took him back into my caseload.

This was not the only time that I encountered unprovoked or unpredictable explosive reactions and *caution* is the only protection.

CONFIRMATION

Believe Nothing

As stated above and in several other places, sex offenders are manipulative and strongly involved in denial, projection and rationalization. Now let us add one further defense mechanism to this list: *Partialization.* I define *partialization* as the persistent and compulsive practice of telling only part of the story. Sex offenders are overly concerned with acceptance and the concomitant fear of rejection. They also want to get the whole process of therapy over as quickly as possible, with the least amount of exposure and pain. Thus it is not uncommon for a therapist to sincerely believe that a client has totally exposed himself, when in reality he has only exposed the outer core of memories, incidents and confessions that he feels comfortable in handling or having the therapist know.

An example will clarify:

☐ PETER *is a 39-year-old, decorated Vietnam veteran who was recently paroled on a rape charge and violated his parole. Upon his return to the treatment program as a violator, he vehemently denied committing the new rape and used all of his savings, his family's assets and even went into considerable debt appealing the charge. No one else doubted Peter's guilt as the rape occurred in broad daylight and the circumstances made identification easy and unmistakable. Still Peter's protestations of innocence and his denial continued for seven years. Late one evening as I was finishing up some paperwork in my office, I received a call that Peter was extremely upset and had to be seen as an emergency referral. When he entered the office, he was on the verge of hysteria, crying, wringing his hands and unable to sit still. He walked around the office in this manner for a while and then regained some composure, sat, and stated "I can't live like this anymore! It's all been a lie! I not only committed that rape but at least six others since I was paroled!"*

While reluctant to explain his seven years of denial he finally admitted that "I'm no good, evil, rotten! I belong locked up for the rest of my life, that's why I raped again!" Due to the degree of his emotional upset, no further probing was possible that evening, but a follow-up session was scheduled for the next day. In a much calmer mood and in control of his emotions, Peter told me that he had been in one of the most notorious Vietnam massacres. He had raped young women in a village at the order of his platoon leader and then took his squad to another village and ordered each member of his group to rape the village leader's wife and daughter, making the father and other village leaders watch. He then, again on orders of his superiors, ordered his men to kill everyone in the village. To this day, he wakes up screaming with nightmares of the incident and cannot find a way to forgive himself.

The importance of Peter in this discussion is that, had this been discovered in his first nine years of therapy, there may not have been another rape victim and he may not have been additionally traumatized by his own behavior. As it now stands, therapy is at a standstill. He wants to do all of the time on his sentence, and were he released, might again rape and possibly kill to assure that he would never be released from prison again.

The Group Confirms Changes and New Behaviors

In Peter's case (as well as hundreds of others), therapists basing their judgments on the client's input would have made terrible errors and effected many more victimizations. In all cases of sex offenders, whether seen in private practice or in an institutional setting, *the therapist is perceived as having total control of the client's life.* Regardless of the situation, ranging from self-report deviant behavior to court- action referrals, the client knows that he has broken the law and can be sent to prison for his deviant acts. Developing the rapport necessary for total trust is difficult at best, and in most cases nearly impossible.

However, where group therapy is concerned, especially in an institutional setting where the clients live, eat and sleep with each other, the group can far better evaluate and judge changes or lack of changes in an individual member of the group.

It must be noted at this juncture that I strongly believe that *behavior is the only real, concrete proof of true therapeutic change.* As stated before, sex offenders, in or out of an institution, are experts at analyzing the wants/needs of therapists. They learn amazingly quickly, by studying the therapist's reactions, comments, follow-up questions, change of subject, body-language, facial expressions, etc., whether their answers, confessions or comments are pleasing or upsetting to the therapist. Wanting to please and desperately needing approval and acceptance, they will then pattern their sessions to gain said approval and acceptance.

There are revelations in this type of therapy that will shock anyone, others that appear comical, others that generate immediate anger and even disgust, if one is not prepared. The therapist needs to maintain a *poker-face*, hiding all personal reactions no matter how difficult this may be.

The Therapist's Comfort with Sexuality

Early in Chapter 9 the reader was asked to identify the most important personal trait that should be a prerequisite to working with offenders. The correct response (from my viewpoint) is *comfort with all aspects of sexuality, in general, and with your own sexuality in particular.* If this condition is met, there will be no prejudgments, no prejudices, no moral imperative or prohibitions and therefore less chance of a shocking revelation damaging the therapeutic process. Whether the revelation involves masturbating an elephant or a dog, licking feces, molestation by a mother, raping 18-month-old babies, or other shocking acts that sex offenders do and need to confess, the therapist who has dealt with his/her own sexual issues will be better equipped to handle the situation without harm to either himself/herself or to the client.

My suggestion for this type of preparation is that all therapists who intend to work with sex offenders or their victims be mandated to attend and participate in an extended S.A.R. (Sex-Attitude-Restructuring) seminar and training session. The desensitization alone that takes place during an S.A.R. is worth the money, time and effort. In an S.A.R., the individual is exposed to a variety of sexually explicit films, several shown simultaneously (depending on the equipment available at the site). In professionally operated S.A.R.'s as many as 12 screens operate at the same time, allowing the participant to watch or to avoid, all significant factors. After each 20 minute film session, the large group divides into small randomly chosen discussion groups. Each subgroup has a facilitator who is very carefully trained in this work. The facilitator guides discussion of the films and the participant's reactions to them and then carefully suggests the possible need for further work or counseling in a particular area.

If taken seriously and honestly, these workshops can offer the participant an opportunity to learn a great deal about himself/herself. *Prejudices, fears, moral indignations, disgusts, turn-ons and turn-offs* can all become quite conscious during both the viewing of the films and also during the discussions that follow. Reacting or overreacting to what is said in the group discussions is extremely important since the same reaction is possible with a client.

Once the trainee/participant has learned facts about his/her sexual values, prejudices, fears, doubts, etc., then he/she can take appropriate remedial measures before treating patients with any form of sexual dysfunction. A personal example will clarify:

☐ *In 1969, I attended a week-long training seminar in California for certification as a sex therapist. Prior to attending the course, I felt that I was more than liberal and that there was nothing sexual that could upset or disturb me. After all, I had been functioning as a sex therapist for at least seven years.*

After a prolonged S.A.R. with 12 screens displaying explicit sexual behavior between consenting adults, the group was asked to fill out evaluation forms, detailing our reactions, preferences, likes and dislikes, etc. When all of the papers were collected, the mentor/facilitator, a motherly, petite female gynecologist (who subsequently was dubbed "Mom"), said to the group: "Now that all of you have lied on the evaluations, who would like to have their paper back and do a new one?" The professionals in the group were highly insulted, myself included, until, from behind each of the 12 screens stepped evaluators who stared at each of us with a clipboard in their hands. They had been watching our reactions during the showing of the films and knew what we avoided, what we didn't want to be seen watching, etc. Without a moment's hesitation, I went forward and asked for my paper back and filled out a new and honest one. Later that evening, in an individual session with an advisor, I was asked only one question: "Why did I lie on the first form?" Was it image or was it fear of facing myself?

Today, I mark that training session as the beginning of my being a true sex therapist. I learned a great deal about myself and had enough material to work on personally and with a colleague for over a year.

Relatives, Staff, and Family as Therapeutic Aides

The group confirmation process can be further enhanced by other outside sources to confirm or deny essential changes in behavior. I have used wives, parent(s), siblings, children (especially in incest), employers, neighbors, personal friends or anyone I could recruit to aid in the treatment of an offender in my private practice. Permission from the client is necessary and I do not divulge any confidences during these contacts. They are simply for information/confirmation and this is made clear from the beginning to both the client and the volunteer.

Simple questioning techniques are utilized that do not contain psychological jargon or diagnostic terminology. Please note that the volunteer must be guaranteed confidentiality, just as the client is, if one is to expect honest and real answers to questions. This applies especially to wives, children and lovers who either fear the client or fear losing the relationship.

A few examples will clarify:

- *"How has ... been doing lately?"*
- *"What is the current status of your relationship with ...?"*
- *"Are you feeling more comfortable talking to ... lately?"*
- For wives/lovers: *"How has sex been the last few weeks with ...?"*
- For children: *"Are you less afraid of your father now than you were or are things still the same?"*
- For employers or co-workers: *"Have you seen any change in ... in the last few weeks? If so, what are they?"*
- For families: *"Are things around the house less tense since ... has been coming to therapy?"*
- For institutional staff: *"Has ... been any different lately? If so, in what way?"* Also: *"Has ... been socializing any more lately than before? If so, with whom and how often?"*

The last question is important since most sex offenders tend to remain isolated in their rooms until changes begin.

All questions should be patterned by the particular circumstances of the case and can be much more directive and pointed than questions used with the offender himself. An example will clarify:

☐ KENNY *had spent five years in therapy for sodomizing teenage boys. His victims were usually hitchhikers whom he picked up, drove to lonely parks or deserted factory areas and then, threatening their lives with a gun, forced them to undress and submit to his sexual assaults. He then drove them home, threatening their families with death if they reported him or told anyone. During five or more years of therapy, he based his insight into his crimes on the sexual abuse he received at the hands of an older stepbrother, who was the parents' favorite and who they would believe in preference to him. His therapeutic progress continued positively as did his behavior. He was a clever young man and everyone tended to be seduced by his wily ways. However, something bothered me about this individual and somehow (gut reaction) I felt we were being conned.*

On a family picnic day, I happened to meet his parents before he arrived at the picnic area and we began to talk. They were interested in his progress and I was positive in my comments to them. By chance I asked how Kenny's stepbrother was doing. The parents looked astounded and remarked that "You must have us confused with another family, since Kenny is an only child. We never had any other children. Kenny always wanted a brother of his own. We spoiled him something awful. He got everything he wanted, except a brother." The other therapists involved with Kenny were just as shocked and astounded as I was. So was his group when I confronted him with the new information. Smiling (or sneering) he admitted that "he had heard the story work before and decided to use it." He never thought anyone would check up on him.

CONTINUATION/CONSISTENCY

Aftercare Is Essential

For offenders who are released from an institutional setting, whether private clinic, hospital or correctional facility, *aftercare by that facility* is essential. In my experience, leaving an institutional setting is, in itself, traumatic for the sex offender. He has become *comfortable,* had few responsibilities, little or no financial problems and has been cared for (food, clothing and shelter) as if by parents. In fact, the institution has become a substitute parent in all these areas, including telling him when to eat, sleep, recreate, etc. In addition, work (if it does exist) is usually foreign to his past experience, and artificial in that it usually lasts only an hour or two per day. Now, he has to again become an independent, self-sufficient person.

For those with families and a home to return to, the transition is much easier. However, there is still a feeling of *strangeness and not belonging* that must be gradually overcome. Finding a job becomes a major problem. For those without family and home, the trauma is even greater. Finding a place to live and a job at the same time appears impossible. The longer the institutional stay, the harder the problem seems to be. For both groups, the first sexual encounter will be frightening (fear of impotence or failure in satisfying a partner) and for the more passive-dependent types, finding relationships at all appears impossible. Thus support in the form of aftercare counseling becomes an essential factor for a successful return to the community.

Emergency Access to the Therapist May Be Necessary

Due to the fears, doubts and exaggerated reactions that the released sex offender experiences, access to his/her own therapist, at least by telephone, is necessary to maintain the gains achieved in the course of treatment. A different therapist or one not acquainted with the forms of treatment he received may say the wrong things and offer suggestions that are new and foreign at a time when continuation and consistency are crucial.

Consistent Treatment Is Important

This access is necessary on a 24-hour basis and both private therapists and institutions must have an "on-call" system or an answering service in place if failure is to be prevented. During vacations, another therapist *totally familiar with the client* should be assigned to handle his/her problems. In institutional settings, this continuation and consistency can be achieved easily if more than one therapist is involved in the case, either as a secondary opinion therapist, an ancillary program therapist or a roaming substitute therapist utilized during illnesses and vacations.

If, upon release, this support must be obtained from a new agency rather than the one from which the offender was released, the task is even more problematic. Most new agencies will want to start therapy all over again, *their way*. Putting the client through his past once again can retrigger the entire problem and often does. I have had released offenders return to me for treatment from as far as two adjoining states because they could not relate to local therapists and did not want to repeat years of painful and guilt-provoking treatment. If the goal of treatment is to integrate the now ex-offender successfully into society and to prevent his victimizing anyone again, these measures, as difficult as they may seem, are necessary and essential.

Sex Offenders Are Never Really "Cured"

Sex offenders are never cured and therefore they may experience recurrences both easily and frequently, at least at the thought and fantasy levels. Treatment (usually in a relapse prevention module) must include making the sex offender recognize this fact, and preparing himself (or herself) to deal with it should it occur. This requires continual contact with the therapist, support individuals and groups in the community. *Prn* status (call in when necessary) in therapy should never be attempted until these factors are adequately covered and internalized.

11

Sexual "Imprinting" as a Consequence of Early Traumatic Molestation

In nearly 30 years of treating males with sexual dysfunction, I have met literally hundreds of clients who have reported instances of *unwanted, disturbing and guilt-provoking behaviors* that could not be explained by their present values, attitudes and/or traumas. There are several different ways in which this phenomenon manifests itself:

- Unwanted sexual reactions/turn-ons
- Self-punishing behaviors
- Negative self-esteem reactions
- Unwanted and unexplained isolation behaviors.

We will consider each one separately for purposes of clarity.

UNWANTED SEXUAL REACTIONS/TURN-ONS

An example may prove helpful:

☐ CHUCK *is a 19-year-old, happily married young man. After a year of hard work, Chuck is given a promotion to a vice-presidency in the corporation where he works. One of his new perks is a membership in an executive health club where he hopes to lose some weight and meet some new friends. The club is great and Chuck is as excited as he's ever been about a new adventure. What makes it even better is*

● COMMON FACTORS FOUND IN IMPRINTING

☐ *1. A Trigger*
☐ *2. An Unwanted Behavior*
☐ *3. A Confusion Reaction*
☐ *4. An Isolation Reaction*
☐ *5. Guilt and Self-Recrimination*
☐ *6. Generalized Sexual Dysfunctions*

that it is a unisex club and he sees many extremely attractive young women that he would like to meet. The first evening goes well: he really enjoys the program of exercises, feels accepted and liked by the other executives. He has already met several new friends of both sexes. Following two hours of happy and hard workouts, the time for his group is up. While the rest of his group goes into the men's locker room to change and shower, Chuck is called to the office to have his picture taken for his identification card. When he arrives in the locker room to change, the rest of the men are in a large open shower and Chuck catches himself staring at their bodies and, in particular, at their genitals. Concurrently, he feels a stirring in his groin and an instant flush of embarrassment, shock and panic occur. He quickly pulls his street clothes over his gym shorts and leaves the health club, sure that he will never return.

At home, Chuck lays on his bed, fear and tears welling up, and replays the mental tapes of what has just occurred. To this point in his life, Chuck remembers only being interested in women and has considered himself a normal 19-year-old heterosexual male. Now, there are doubts. In a few weeks, he becomes aware of ancillary, strange new behaviors: he is avoiding any possible male contacts; he no longer uses the urinals at work but locks himself into a booth instead; he finds excuses and alibis to get out of any possible male-oriented social gatherings (such as stopping for a few beers after work). Finally, the next time (after the incident) that his wife initiates sex, he is totally impotent. After almost six months of this hell, Chuck calls for an appointment and slowly and painfully exposes the incident, his fears and his present state of isolation, anxiety and impotence.

This same type of scenario has been heard from girls and women, high school boys, scoutmasters, ministers and priests as well as other individuals from all professions and walks of life. Let's look at another example:

☐ MIKE, *introduced in Chapter 6, has been married for almost ten years and his wife has just had the beautiful son he has always hoped and prayed for. Mike is a lieutenant in the Navy Reserve and is in line for promotion to captain. He has had many happy and successful working and socializing experiences with men, without problems. He is well-liked and highly sociable. Being community-minded, he also is a scout leader and has been on several camping trips with a group of scouts. Shortly following his wife's return from the hospital with their new baby son, Mike's wife asked him to help her give the baby a bath and he willingly and excitedly agreed. While he held and washed his infant son, he caught himself staring at the baby's penis and felt himself becoming excited. He instantly fantasized touching and fondling his son's penis and wanting to* make his son "feel good" *in that manner.*

Like Chuck, he panicked, yelled for his wife and made the excuse that he feared hurting or dropping the baby. She took over and he left the room in a state of fear, tension and confusion. From that moment on, Mike's life changed dramatically: at work, he waited until all of the other officers had showered and were in bed before doing so himself; he copped-out of the upcoming hunting trip with several of his friends that he had been looking forward to for several months. He desperately tried to get out of taking his scouts on a scheduled camp-out but could not, so with trepidation, he went (the only adult on the trip).

The first night, after all the scouts were asleep, he stayed awake until two or three A.M., torturing himself with the memory of what had happened with his son. Glancing over at the sleeping boys, he noticed that one of the boys, SCOTT, had kicked off his blankets and went over to cover him. When he arrived at the bunk, he was startled to see that Scott was exposed and had a rigid erection in his sleep. Without hesitation he knelt by the bed and began to masturbate Scott, his only thought being to bring the boy to his first orgasm and ejaculation. He did just that and it appeared that Scott had slept through the entire incident. Mike covered him up and left the area to torture himself again with recriminations. His fears were well-founded. The evening after returning home two policemen arrived at Mike's home with a warrant for his arrest. Scott had been awake. Due to his excellent record in the community, he was permitted diversion with the agreement of immediate treatment, and that is when I first met him.

Finally, let us take a look at a case involving a woman.

☐ MARY, *age 31, was a very attractive, intelligent single woman with several degrees. At the time of her referral, she was functioning as a supervisor in a mental health agency that supervised a great many adolescent clients. Mary's primary complaint was that she was anorgasmic. She had recently met and been dating a younger man, ANDY, age 26, who was getting impatient with her excuses for not "going all the way" and she feared losing him. One evening, after an hour or more of heavy petting, Andy finally gave her an ultimatum, stating the suspicion that "maybe something is wrong with you." He took her home and promised to call. The call never came.*

At about the same time, a new employee was assigned to her department: a young, attractive and openly friendly young woman towards whom Mary felt attracted. She found excuses to work more and more closely with the new woman and began touching her on the shoulder, rubbing her neck or back, etc. The woman responded warmly and gratefully. Mary felt strange feelings and panicked. She withdrew from any contact with the young woman and concentrated on dating Andy. In the next week or so, Mary noticed several changes in both her personality and her behavior: she became less assertive and had difficulty making decisions; she isolated herself from most of her friends and all of her social activities; and she began to feel more and more attracted to her female supervisees, while avoiding prolonged contact with her male supervisees.

In the third or fourth week, she began feeling *erotic* toward the females and panicked. This is when she made her first appointment, deciding *not* to tell the real reason for coming to a sex therapist.

COMMON FACTORS FOUND IN THE THREE CASES

In each of the three cases illustrated above, there were several common factors:

The Trigger

This is usually a behavior or event that, before it occurred, was seen or considered to be normal, happy, positive, etc. In Chuck's case, it was his joining the health club; in Mike's case, it was finally having the son he wanted and dreamed of; in Mary's case, it was falling in love with Andy and being rejected.

It should be noted that the *trigger* could be a traumatic event as well, especially if it duplicated the original imprinting cause. This will be explained more fully later.

The Unwanted Behavior

This is usually an act or reaction, *always* with a physical component, that is totally out of the ordinary for the individual and, to his conscious memory, has never occurred before. In Chuck s case, it consisted of staring at the genitals of the men in the showers and becoming sexually excited; in Mike's case, it consisted of wanting to touch his son's penis and later, and even more unwanted, his sexual molestation of one of his scouts; and in Mary's case, it consisted of becoming interested in her new female supervisee in an erotic way.

A Confusion Reaction

Immediately following the first incident of the unwanted behavior, a sense of bewilderment and confusion occurs. This is primarily due to the fact that the behavior *makes no sense* to the individual experiencing it, and does not seem to fit or belong in the individual's life. For example in Chuck's case, the bewilderment and confusion he felt when he became aware that he was staring at the other men's genitals and felt the stirring in his groin. In Mike's case, his confusion over the desires and fantasies of touching his son's penis and giving him pleasure through fondling it. In Mary's case, her confusion involved feeling erotic toward her young female supervisee, since she had supervised many other women for many years without such a reaction or feeling.

An Isolation Reaction

In all cases observed to date, an isolation reaction was seen and is considered an avoidance or escape behavior to prevent a second or more disastrous occurrence. All of the clients treated paranoidally predicted that the next incident would increase the depth or severity of unwanted behavior, usually, as in Mike's case, involving acting out the impulse, fantasy or desire. This reaction is dramatic and, although the clients continue to work daily and normally, in most, if not all instances, their social contacts and behaviors are dramatically eliminated from their lifestyle.

Guilt and Self-Recriminations

In all the cases I have seen over the past 30 years, *guilt* was the major reaction to such unwanted behaviors. The guilt produced damaging behavior as well as a negative self-image, feelings of abnormality and a dangerous destruction of self-esteem. More than one of these clients had contemplated suicide and several had actually gone so far as to have made an attempt before seeking professional help.

Generalized Sexual Dysfunctions

In each of the cases seen, there were abrupt changes in sexual functioning. This is usually the reported reason for seeking sex therapy. These changes include *inversion* of the former sexual identity, *paraphilic* behaviors, and *desire-phase* problems accompanied by abstinence. Even masturbation may now pose a threat.

QUESTIONS ABOUT ETIOLOGY

After experiencing several hundred cases of this type, a theoretical hypothesis was developed to try to explain the *imprinting* phenomenon and to help create a treatment model for those patients in severe distress. The hypothesis was:

> *The first pleasurable orgasm in an individual's life imprints and will remain with that individual in some form for the remainder of his/her life, either consciously or unconsciously.*

In each case where the imprinting phenomenon was observed, therapy uncovered an early long-term (versus single occurrence) sexual seduction that was at least initially experienced as *positive*. This, in itself, does not explain the imprinting since, were this a traumatic and negative-affect experience, a different reaction would have been expected. The imprint appears dependent on a *positive-affect situation* — one where the sexual seduction occurred in a positive way with many benefits attached: affection, love (paraphilic), both emotional and material support (clothes, trips, movies, physical contact, a port-in-the-storm, a parental substitute and a myriad of other benefits that the child wanted or needed).

A relationship developed that was *perceived* as positive and beneficial until exposure or separation occurred. Where exposure of the abuse occurred in a *positive* manner, no trauma need occur but the imprint will remain and needs to be explained and dealt with in therapy, as soon as possible. Where exposure of the abuse occurred in a *negative* manner, that trauma in itself often results in a partial or total *repression* of the event or a *delusional distortion,* especially if the seduction occurred in late childhood or early adolescence. This is often precipitated by one or more adults involved in negatively reacting to the exposure. The child then either represses the event totally or changes the reality of the occurrence and adds threat, fear, pressure, etc., that in reality did not exist. A caveat: this only *explains* the behavior, it does not *justify* it.

Years may pass, even an entire developmental stage, where no conscious memory of the relationship exists and the child develops along accepted, normal pathways. Let us now see how this theoretical framework fits into our three example cases:

☐ *In Chuck's case, the early seduction was begun at age 11 by a teacher in junior high school. Chuck was a sensitive, quiet, well-behaved boy who did well in most of his subjects but had trouble with mathematics. His father had deserted the family early in Chuck's life and his mother worked, sometimes two jobs, to keep the family going. The teacher picked Chuck as a potential victim almost from the first day of the new school year. Within a month, he had assigned Chuck as class monitor, given him special after school jobs and offered to tutor him in math at his apartment, if his mother consented. The attention Chuck was receiving was everything he had wanted from his missing father and he literally couldn't get enough. Chuck easily convinced his mother to allow the personal tutoring and, little by little, the teacher introduced private and special games into their weekend meetings. The games began with strip- poker, progressed to measuring penises, then to discussions of sex and finally into sex education that resulted in the teacher masturbating Chuck to explain erection, orgasm and ejaculation. When Chuck could not ejaculate, at first, the teacher had Chuck masturbate him in order to complete the lesson. Oral sex came next and became their usual sexual activity, often as a reward for excellent homework or for doing well in a tutored lesson.*

This relationship lasted for Chuck's final year of junior high school. He then left for a different school in another part of town. There he met other budding teenagers and joined their activities. Within those three years of senior high school, Chuck had his first heterosexual encounter, a train (another name for a gang sexual experience, where the newest or youngest boy is last in line) that he enjoyed. From then on, until the incident at 19, his sexual behavior was heterosexual and the relationship with the teacher was forgotten (repressed). Being nude in the health club locker room with other adult men triggered a forgotten erotic impulse and the unwanted behavior occurred. The memory remained repressed hence the confusion, anxiety, etc., and the need for therapeutic intervention.

☐ *In Mike's case, the scenario differed only in the cast. The seducer was a roomer that his mother had taken in to help pay the bills after his father died. The roomer slept nude in the same room with Mike and one night slid into Mike's bed, suggested that Mike also sleep nude and then reached over, fondled him and masturbated him. Mike was either ten or eleven at the time and the relationship lasted until he was 13. Mike liked his new friend and they went camping, fishing, etc. The roomer supplied whatever Mike wanted that his mother could not afford. When the roomer moved out, Mike missed him but then began associating more with his peer group. He was subsequently initiated into the wonders of the opposite sex, lost his virginity and remained heterosexual in interest, fantasy and behavior until the birth of his long-awaited son. Even after the incident while bathing his son, he did not remember the roomer.*

It took six months of therapy before the early memories finally began to emerge; slowly at first and then like a raging waterfall. What was amazing was the depth and the detail that emerged. Once the barrier was broken, memories of words, phrases, feelings, even smells emerged. The most important memory was that when Mike asked the roomer why he was masturbating him, the roomer answered "to make you feel good," later tied in with "because I love you."

☐ *Finally, Mary, a slightly different case. Seduction by an aunt when she began menstruating, clitoral stimulation to the point of pain and a horrifying day when her mother was observed watching them naked in bed, were all factors that emerged in the course of therapy. The last one — being caught by her mother — resulted in a plethora of curses, slurs, putdowns and name calling that ended in Mary being blamed for what the aunt (the mother's sister) had initiated.*

Sex for Mary was labeled as sinful, dirty, evil, the invention of Satan, etc., and Mary was forbidden to ever touch herself there again. As time passed, Mary also repressed this incident but not the admonitions about sex. Although still not remembered (her memories returned periodically in small spurts) there must have also been a warning about men and sex with men. Mary is still unable to tolerate seeing pictures of a naked man for even a split second, nor can she view sexually-explicit movies. Therapy will continue for quite some time.

THERAPEUTIC CONSIDERATIONS AND CAVEATS

Naturally, the first therapeutic goal of import is to discover the early event(s) that imprinted and eventually triggered the unwanted behavior. Usually, this has been found to be an early sexual seduction that was positive and pleasant over a period of time and that for some reason, traumatic or not, was totally repressed for quite a number of years.

Once the event(s) is totally uncovered and all the emotions, labeling, and revulsion have been ventilated, the therapist can proceed therapeutically as with any recent survivor of a sexual seduction. The ambivalent feelings about the seducer in the story must be thoroughly explored and accepted. Often religion, parental values, societal values and personal belief systems are at play and need to be thoroughly explored and dealt with as well.

Next, sex-attitude-restructuring becomes a paramount concern. By now, where *inversion* is concerned, the client has labeled himself/herself "queer," "abnormal," etc. In reality, these confused individuals are *bisexual* and must be made to understand that accepting this fact (which I believe is unalterable due to the imprinting) does not mean that they ever have to act out in this manner. Thus Chuck, while he may catch himself sexually attracted to or stimulated by men, can remain heterosexual behaviorally and never become involved in a homosexual act.

Individuals with imprinting problems containing inversion elements feel and believe that once they experience sexual stimulation from a same-sex person, that eventually *they must act on it.* This is not the case.

☐ *Once Chuck accepted this fact, he was able to return to the health club, have similar reactions to the original unwanted behavior, but not panic or leave. He has become accustomed to these reactions and is no longer threatened or concerned about them. His former social life has been reactivated, and he has become more sensitive to other men's needs and can even be socially physical (hugging, horseplay, wrestling, etc.) with them without a problem. He is no longer important and his sex life with his wife has been described by both as "fantastic!" He has been out of therapy now for about a year.*

☐ *Mike, since he committed a sexual offense, remains in therapy on a monthly basis at the order of the court and will continue for at least another year or more. At that time, he can appeal to the court to terminate therapy. Sex with his wife is back to normal (they both went through a complete sex therapy course that they needed badly). Mike can now change and bathe his son without problems, although his wife must be present by court demand. Masturbation fantasies, at rare times, include memories of himself and the roomer, but they are pleasant and erotic. While presently not interested in a male-male encounter, he does not preclude the possibility in the future and has discussed this with his wife, who accepts it "as long as it does not contain love" (her condition).*

☐ *Mary, however, although she understands and accepts what happened to her and the imprint it left, is still in therapy. Progress has been made on a work level where she again is able to function well as a supervisor with both sexes. Her social life remains minimal with no man in her life at present. She has not decided whether she wants to work in that area or to "leave things as they are since it is safe" (her words). As with all clients, the decision is hers and only time will tell what she will choose. She accepts her bisexual thoughts with little or no guilt but remains sexually inactive. She is learning to masturbate and has had success in becoming orgasmic.*

CONCLUSIONS AND FUTURE CONSIDERATIONS

In this chapter, I have discussed only our experiences with positive imprinting where sexually unwanted behavior is concerned. I have also observed unwanted guilt behaviors based on negative imprinting from extremely restrictive, punishing experiences in childhood and adolescence, especially those associated with incest. The results of these negative forms of imprinting are just as disastrous as those involving the sexually unwanted behaviors resulting from positive imprinting.

Treatment is identical for both forms. First, identify the imprint cause and then begin treatment as with a survivor of sexual abuse at an early age and/or exposure. While often a painful and difficult treatment process, the majority of cases are successful, and adjustment is oriented to the goals that the patient/client sets. Specialized techniques are involved and we repeat our caveat to our colleagues that they should not attempt these cases without special training and supervised experience.

IMPRINTING IN SEX OFFENDERS

Where sex offenders are concerned, an interesting phenomenon has been observed that takes on *ritualistic* overtones. I have found this pattern of ritual in both pedophiles and hebophiles. Choice of victim type, sex and age, choice of setting for the act and choice of specific sex act all appear to be determined by the imprint made at the offender's own victimization or sexual seduction. An example will clarify.

☐ AL *was arrested for sexual molestation of six-and seven-year-old neighborhood boys. The offenses followed this pattern: he would lure the child into his garage where there was nothing except a single chair near a workbench. In the* first *occurrence with each child, he would sit the child on his lap for a few seconds and then tell him to go home. In the* second *occurrence, he would sit the child on his lap and rub his back. In the* third *occurrence, he would sit the child on his lap, rub his back and extend the rubbing into the child's pants in order to rub his buttocks. In the* fourth *occurrence, he would sit the child on his lap, rub his* back, extend the rubbing into the child's pants in order to rub his buttocks and then reach around the front to fondle his genitals and masturbate him.

This ritualistic behavior occurred with three boys before a fourth boy reported the incident to his parents, whereupon Al was arrested and sent for treatment. Therapy over a six-month period revealed no pedophilic fantasies and no homosexual thoughts or occurrences. While he denied any conscious memory of being molested as a child, there was a total absence of any memories for the period around age six. Memories before and after this age were as expected. Finally, hypnosis was utilized and on the third hypnotic regression the following story unfolded.

Al, age six, lived next door to a bachelor who had a toy shop in his garage. Al would hang around the open garage door watching, in fascination, the tinkering and seemingly magical production of toys for the next Christmas season. Finally, the toymaker invited Al in and the following episodes occurred during his next four visits: On the first visit: the toymaker sat Al on his lap; on the second visit, the toymaker sat Al on his lap and rubbed back; on the third visit, the toymaker sat Al on his lap, rubbed his back, went into his pants and rubbed his buttocks; on the fourth visit, the toymaker sat Al on his lap, rubbed his back, went into his pants, rubbed his buttocks and then moved to the front and fondled his genitals and masturbated him. This went on for over a year, unreported, and then, without explanation, the toymaker moved.

This exact repetition of the details and events of an original molestation that is later repressed has been seen in literally hundreds of offenders over the last quarter of a century.

If asked why a specific age range is targeted (e.g., 7-9, 9-11, 12-14, 15-17) the most frequent response is "They're the best!" or an equivalent phrase with a similar meaning. If asked why a specific choice of act (e.g., fondling versus oral or anal sex) the response is "That's the one I like best!" or "That one feels best to me!" or some equivalent response.

We have actually, on many occasions, had arguments in groups of pedophiles and hebophiles as to what age, physical build, hair color, body type, act, etc., is best. The *imprint effect* extends also to the place or setting of the seduction/molestation. For example, if their own experience had been in the woods or on a camping trip, this will be the setting they choose for seducing their victims; if in an attic or cellar, that will be their choice of setting; if in a garage (as with Al) this will be the preferred setting.

In some one hundred offenders queried (regardless of sex or age of victim), this phenomenon was observed and verified in over 90% of the cases. The remaining ten percent had multiple seduction/molestations, all of different types, with different individuals and with a variety of sex acts. With these offenders, the imprint effect held only for age group and male/female choice.

OFFENDER PATTERNS

The following sequence appears to occur in sex offenders:

- An early sexual seduction occurs that is not discovered or reported and that contains a pleasurable orgasm and also other pleasant elements such as friendship, gifts, money, caring, trips, etc.

- The relationship ends abruptly either because the offender moves, the child moves, the child changes schools, etc. This leaves an emotional scarring that leads to or results in a total *repression* of any of the events of the relationship until many years later.

- A *trigger* event occurs and the behavior is reactivated with a *role reversal*: the former victim now becomes the adult victimizer with a child victim who is the same age as he was at the time of his own molestation. For Mike this was the birth of his son; for Chuck it was the sight of all the naked men in the health club shower and his becoming stimulated.

- Thoughts and fantasies containing the desire to *reenact* the former scenario begin, sometimes instantly, from the onset of the trigger event. While, at first, these are *obsessive* thoughts and fantasies, they then translate into *compulsive* behavior over which the offender claims little or no control, regardless of the severity of the consequences. Teachers, for example, know they will never be allowed to teach again; husbands fear divorce; all fear exposure and prison, but they do not stop (nor can they). When finally caught and arrested, there is a sense of relief that is openly expressed early in the treatment process.

- Immediate *behavioral changes* occur: flight, guilt and social isolation being the most frequently observed and reported. Chuck ran out of the health club vowing never to return and avoiding all social contact, especially with males; Mike ran out of the baby's room and never again would participate in either changing the baby's diaper or bathing him; Chuck became impotent with his wife; Mike stopped having sex with his wife; Mary stopped dating men.

PREVENTION

Prevention appears dependent on reporting or some form of disclosure at the age that the seduction/molestation occurred. I interviewed 25 men, molested at an early age, who had reported the event and received either short-term therapy or were given adequate explanations to handle the associated fear, guilt, etc. The main personality difference in these men, when compared to sex offenders, was that they did not put the blame or guilt on themselves, but rather on the offender, where it belonged. Their self-

- **FACTORS IN ABUSED CHILDREN WHO DID NOT REPORT AND WHO DID NOT BECOME SEX OFFENDERS AS ADULTS**

  ☐ 1. Their self-esteem was strong and positive.

  ☐ 2. They had a fairly good sexual knowledge at the time of the molestation/seduction.

  ☐ 3. There was an important adult in their lives with whom they could discuss anything without fear of repercussion.

  ☐ 4. Their religious education was along positive and forgiving pathways.

  ☐ 5. They had several real friends in their peer group with whom they could discuss anything.

  ☐ 6. Their personality structure was stronger and more positive than the usually quite inadequate sex offender.

  ☐ 7. They were successful in school, sports or some other area that produced pride, both for their parents and themselves.

  ☐ 8. Their parents were more regularly involved in their lives and activities, attended P.T.A.'s and other school functions, and spent as much time as possible with them on weekends, etc. They also traveled and vacationed with their parents.

  ☐ 9. They believed in themselves and had large amounts of self-confidence.

  ☐ 10. They were long-term-goal oriented in contrast to the living-day-by-day lifestyle of the sex offender.

esteem remained intact. They did not change their sexual identity or orientation because of the molestation. On the whole, they were able to accept the benefits (whether the sexual pleasure, the gifts, the relationship, etc.) without feeling that *they caused the molestation* as other traumatized victims do, as in the following types of perceptions:

- "I must have been seductive or too pretty or turned him on."
- "My body was too nice or too sexual and caused him to do what he did."

The survivors' lives remain unaltered and their development continues along normal lines. From this group, I learned several important preventive factors that were part of their lives and not part of the usual sex offender's life. The importance of a list of such factors is obvious: *If these strengths and educational elements can be incorporated into the lives of all of our children, then the sex offenders will have less chance of success, except by force.* Note that not all ten factors were present in all 25 men interviewed; however, there were at least six of the ten factors present in all of the test group.

The importance of these ten factors (and there may be more) is that they clearly indicate that *if* children could be brought up in a more positive environment and *if* parents could be educated to *accentuate the positives and minimize or utilize the negatives,* fewer children would be so readily available to the child molesters.

Since the molesters themselves experienced negativism, hypercritical appraisal and judgment, and a persistent emphasis on their failings and deficiencies, they know all too well the emotional devastation that results and the tremendous need that is generated for acceptance and love *at any price.* These simple changes could greatly reduce the ever-increasing number of children, especially boys, who are being molested and have nowhere to go and no one to trust or confide in. The numbers of sexually disturbed or dysfunctional adults that exist in today's world attests to this problem.

12

Pedophiles: Background and Characteristics

Of the three principal types of sex offenders (pedophiles/hebophiles, rapists, and incestuous fathers), the pedophile is the most complicated and the most difficult to treat. It should also be noted that the number of child molestations has been steadily increasing. A careful study of this particular group may afford the opportunity of preventing this increase from getting even greater, since this deviation is *always* traced back to some form of sexual seduction or trauma in the individual's childhood (see Chapter 2). Therefore, it appears quite logical and appropriate to infer that, *were these childhood sexual traumas discovered at the time they occurred and immediately treated and resolved by trained and competent counselors or therapists, the number of child sexual molestations would eventually decrease rather than continue to increase.*

Broadly defined, adult pedophiles and hebophiles are individuals who prefer, need, and are compulsively drawn to children and adolescents. Among many others who have addressed the topic, Dr. Nicholas Groth has followed the distinction between fixated and regressed pedophiles introduced by Krafft-Ebbing. My own experience confirms Dr. Groth's typology but with the caveat that

♦ A SCHEMATIC REPRESENTATION OF FIXATED VS. REGRESSED PEDOPHILIA: SOURCES, DYNAMICS, OFFENSE CHARACTERISTICS

FIXATED

♦ 1. Primary sexual orientation is to children.

♦ 2. Pedophilic interests begin at adolescence.

♦ 3. No precipitating stress; no subjective distress.

♦ 4. Persistent interest + compulsive behavior.

♦ 5. Pre-planned, premeditated offense.

♦ 6. "Equalization" is the principal dynamic: Offender identifies closely with the victim and "equalizes" his behavior to the level of the child; offender is a "pseudo-peer" to the victim.

♦ 7. Most offenders are single and have little or no sexual contact with age-mates — although some may simultaneously have contact with an age-mate of his own sex, usually serving as a substitute for a child partner, with this interaction typically [mutually] stimulated by the use of child pornography.

♦ 8. Usually no history of alcohol or drug abuse.

♦ 9. Evidence of characterological immaturity with poor socio-sexual peer relationships.

♦ 10. The offense is a maladaptive resolution of life issues.

REGRESSED

♦ 1. Primary sexual orientation is to age-mates.

♦ 2. Pedophilic interests emerge in adulthood.

♦ 3. Precipitating stress is typically evident.

♦ 4. Involvements may be more episodic.

♦ 5. Initial offense is often impulsive rather than premeditated.

♦ 6. "Substitution" is the principal dynamic: Offender replaces conflictual adult relationship[s] with involvement with the child [or with children]; the victim is a "pseudo-adult" substitute.

♦ 7. Sexual contact with children proceeds alongside sexual contact with age-mates; the offender is usually married or living in a common-law [heterosexual] relationship.

♦ 8. In a high proportion of cases, the offense may be alcohol-abetted.

♦ 9. The life-style is more nearly traditional, but with underdeveloped peer relationships.

♦ 10. The offense is a maladaptive attempt to cope with specific life stresses.

not all of the characteristics listed for each classification are always present.

In the simplest of definitions, the *fixated* pedophile has never had an adult sexual experience but *fixated* in psychosexual development in childhood; the *regressed* pedophile, on the other hand, progressed psychosexually into adulthood but when strong, sexual stress was encountered, *regressed* to an earlier psychosexual stage, usually in early to mid adolescence. The primary importance of distinguishing between fixated and regressed pedophilia or hebophilia is for establishing the prognosis for safety and/or the ability to release the offender from institutionalization or community treatment.

The following are the characteristics of *fixated* pedophiles.

- Harder to treat due to their incredible resistance to change.
- They are convinced, as a group, that what they are doing is good for the children and tend to rationalize their behavior in any way possible. They are supported by international organizations like the North American Man-Boy Love Association (NAMBLA) and the Pedophile Information Exchange (PIE), as well as Greek mythology, sociological studies and several prominent psychologists and sexologists, making the therapist's attempts to help them change even more difficult.
- They are much more inadequate than the hebophiles, rapists or incestuous fathers and therefore are less likely to believe that, for them, change is possible.
- They have never had an adult or peer sexual experience and:

    a. Don't want one since they are convinced that they have found the best sexual world of all;

    b. Are terrified of sex with a peer adult since they negatively perceive themselves as inferior in all areas when compared with their peer group;

    c. Are failure-phobic and thus take fewer risks or attempts at new behaviors than the other groups;

    d. By the time they are exposed and either incarcerated or mandated to treatment, they have been actively pedophilic for a great many years and are comfortable in their deviation (happily-maladjusted).

- Their personality-deficits are far more numerous than any of the other groups of offenders and they are aware of this factor.

The *regressed* pedophiles, on the other hand, have much more going for them in the way of positive therapeutic factors:

- They are usually much more guilt-ridden and thus less resistant to change.
- They realize that what they did was wrong and that they harmed their victim(s).
- They are less inadequate than the fixated group and find it easier to believe that change is possible.
- They have had peer/adult sexual relationships and then regressed. Therefore they know that they are capable of adult sexual behavior.
- They have fewer personality deficits than the fixated group and therefore their prognosis is much more positive.

From the above discussion, one can see that differential diagnosis with the overall group of child molesters is essential before any treatment plan can be formulated. After working with the above differentiation, I quickly came to the conclusion that a second delineation was necessary, based on the victim age-group preference. This need arose when, in several groups of exclusively child molesters, I discovered that not only did they disagree with each other on age- choice, but also that their overall personalities were grossly different. The result was the differentiation explained in the next section.

PEDOPHILES VERSUS HEBOPHILES

An important distinction involving child-molesters is that of the *pedophilic* versus the *hebophilic* personality and makeup. On the simplest level, pedophiles are interested in:

- pre-pubertal, non orgasmic children of either sex;
- young children whom they can mold sexually into the rituals that most satisfy their needs; and
- young, weak, easily led and intimidated children whom the offender can easily control and from whom there would be no fear of physical injury.

Hebophiles on the other hand are interested in:

- post-pubertal, orgasmic pre-teens or teenagers who are capable of enjoying sex to orgasm;

• A SCHEMATIC COMPARISON OF PEDOPHILES VS. HEBOPHILES: SOURCES, DYNAMICS, OFFENSE CHARACTERISTICS

PEDOPHILES	HEBOPHILES
◆ 1. Victim age preference: pre-pubertal, anorgasmic.	◆ 1. Victim age preference: post-pubertal, orgasmic.
◆ 2. Age bracket choice depends on the level of inadequacy. A general rule is that the more inadequate the offender, the younger the child victim.	◆ 2. Age bracket choice usually reflects the age at which he was happiest sexually and otherwise. This may be considered his age of psychosexual fixation.
◆ 3. Offender is usually fixated.	◆ 3. Offender is usually regressed. This group includes the incestuous fathers.
◆ 4. Offender's need is to please the child sexually for acceptance. Often uses "sex education" as a ploy.	◆ 4. Offender's need is to have a sex partner. Considers his behavior as "having an affair."
◆ 5. The sexual behavior is usually one-sided with the offender "pleasing" the child victim.	◆ 5. The sexual behavior is usually two-sided with reciprocation a need of the offender.
◆ 6. Gross immaturity and inadequacy prevail.	◆ 6. This group usually is more mature with a good adult facade.
◆ 7. Employment goals are usually below potential. This group prefers passive and subservient positions.	◆ 7. Employment goals are age and potential oriented. This group often contains professionals and successful business men.
◆ 8. Socially, this group fears both their peers as well as adults. They are comfortable only with other inadequate males or children.	◆ 8. Socially, this group gets along well with peers on most levels except sexually.
◆ 9. Treatment time is usually a long-term battle for the smallest, visible or observable changes.	◆ 9. Treatment time usually reflects rapid growth; changes appear sooner and are more easily observed or proven.
◆ 10. Prognosis is extremely poor. This group comprises the most failures of all sex offender groups in treatment.	◆ 10. Prognosis is good. There are more strengths to work with and the success rate is relatively high.

- easily led or influenced youth of either sex who can be controlled and who pose no physical threat; and

- sex partners with whom they can have an affair and yet with whom they cannot live, thereby avoiding the risk of failure in a relationship.

The two groups are vastly different and their prognoses for successful treatment are just as different. The *pedophiles* have the poorest prognosis of all the sex offenders. Many individuals in this group have never had a successful adult sexual relationship but are rather *fixated* at a pre-teen or teenage level of psychosexual development. This group contains the largest number of treatment failures, regardless of approach or environment. The *hebophiles* on the other hand, have usually reached an adult, peer level of sexual relationship but then, due to some real or perceived trauma, *regressed* to a former age level where they were the happiest and safest (usually in the teenage years). This group has a much more positive prognosis and a larger number of rapid successes. The two groups also differ in *personality makeup and characteristics* as can be seen in the schematic comparison of pedophiles vs. hebophiles.

PEDOPHILES VERSUS INCESTUOUS FATHERS

Since *incest* usually involves either children or adolescents, it is necessary and appropriate at this juncture to see the difference between these two groups. While pedophiles differ greatly from incestuous fathers, as can be seen in the schematic comparison chart for the two groups, there is less of a distinction between incestuous fathers and hebophiles. In fact, most incestuous fathers are either regressed pedophiles or hebophiles, but the reverse is not true. Here again, the differential diagnosis aids in determining the individual's overall treatment plan and also is essential for proper and safe prognoses. It is safe to state that the incestuous fathers group has the best prognosis of all the sex offenders and is the easiest and fastest to treat.

THE KING OF THE CASTLE SYNDROME

The major distinguishing characteristic of the incestuous father is his driving and all-pervasive need to function as *"The king of the castle"* in his home. He controls and dominates the lives of his wife and children and rules with an iron hand, oblivious to his own hypocrisy and double standards.

In contrast to the pedophile, he is usually quite socially adept, assertive in work and relational situations, makes friends outside the home easily and has the facade of the most wonderful person on earth. His *secret* home life is unknown to his relatives, including his parents, and his friends. When he is exposed, it is not uncommon for employers, fellow workers and others in the community (often including the authorities) to disbelieve the complaint and to support the offender quite strongly.

The incestuous father often works or volunteers in the community and is awarded the highest honors and praise for his work. Many in this group of offenders have important and responsible positions and many others are self-employed.

An example at this point will clarify:

☐ DONNY *and* JUDY *lived in an upper- middle-class home. Their father,* ALAN, *was a prominent physician and surgeon, well-known in the community and active in child abuse functions on both a local and state level. Unfortunately, Alan was a Jekyll and Hyde personality who ruled his home as a dictator.*

Alan began his incestuous molestations and sadistic, brutal physical abuse of both children when they were approximately seven years old. One particular incident became a crucial traumatic event, the first of many, for Judy. After returning home from a social affair that the whole family attended, Alan took Judy into the living room, undressed her and attempted intercourse with her. Judy was only seven years old. During this molestation, Judy's mother came into the living room, catching Alan in the act. By the utmost denial process, she slapped Judy, called her a "tramp and a whore" and accused her of seducing her father and trying to steal her husband away.

Imagine the impact on a seven year old. From that day on, Judy's mother rejected her totally and wouldn't even speak to her. Shortly afterwards, the mother left the home and the children with the "Monster," as Judy came to identify her father (quite appropriately). Alan now had the children to himself, with no fear of being caught or stopped in his perverse behavior.

Judy now became the woman of the house and from that day on she acted as hostess and sex partner for her father, replacing her mother, although unwillingly. Although there were four children (two other brothers), Judy was closest to Donny and learned years later that Donny also was being sexually molested as well as physically abused by their father. The physical abuse was the most sadistic that I have encountered (outside of sex-mutilation murders). Alan forced absolute submission to his will and punished the children in horrible and sadistic ways, resulting in permanent physical damage. Where Judy was concerned, he forced objects into her vagina, beat her with his fists and objects like baseball bats or whatever else was available. Then he forced her to perform any and all forms of sexual acts, ranging from the normal to the most perverse.

As a result, Judy sustained multiple concussions, since he primarily hit her over the head. He would then take her to the emergency room of the hospital where he practiced and tell the attending physician that: "she's a klutz and accident prone and fell down the stairs again and again and again!" The physicians and hospital staff accepted his stories, or more likely protected the great and mighty physician. This went on until Judy was age 15, when she finally ran away from home and was forced to live and survive on the streets of a major city. To this day, the damage done by her father plagues her with a glandular malfunction.

As for Donny, the same pattern emerged. The extent of Alan's brutality knew no bounds and one night, when Donny had not cooperated to the extent Alan wished, cut his penis nearly off. Donny refused to go to the emergency room with this trauma and Judy helped him to clean and bandage the damaged organ with butterfly stitches, etc. Now they knew that they both were being used.

They also discovered that the monster, Alan, had played them against each other, knowing of their love and affection for each other. If either one balked at his demands, Alan would threaten to go to the other one to get compliance. To defend their sibling, both gave in on such occasions.

While Judy fought and ran away from home when she no longer could bear living that way, Donny could no longer live the life of a forced male prostitute and committed suicide. The shock for Judy almost pushed her into a psychotic break but her inner strengths (that she never recognized) kept her going. She finally made up her mind to confront her father and, if necessary, expose him to the world. Unfortunately, Alan had a major coronary and died before this was possible, leaving a distraught and broken Judy to survive. Her other two brothers wanted to know nothing about what happened to her since they left home as quickly as they were able to and, through extensive denial, were able to mitigate their guilt for not helping either their sister or their brother. Fortunately, Judy has grown and matured on her own to the point where she is now a teacher and soon will finish her education. She then plans to function in some form of crisis counseling, for which she has a natural talent.

Fear and terror tactics on the part of their father, as well as intense shame and guilt for the years of perverted sex with him, prevented either child from reporting him. In addition, Alan convinced them that they would never be believed (a typical incestuous parent ploy), and Judy had had enough hospitalizations to see that the doctors believed (or acted as if they believed) her father. This case clearly points up the divergence in outcome of these cases and also clearly indicates that *the personality strengths and character of the child victim definitely affect the outcome of the case, especially where incest is concerned.*

● A SCHEMATIC COMPARISON OF PEDOPHILES VS. INCESTUOUS FATHERS

PEDOPHILES

♦ 1. These offenders have usually never had a successful adult sexual relationships.

♦ 2. Inadequacy dominates in the group and they fail persistently.

♦ 3. These offenders lose their jobs frequently. They have no direction in their lives and few or no realistic goals.

♦ 4. This group has few, if any, real relationships and they tend to isolate from social interaction.

♦ 5. These offenders are socially inept primarily due to their pervasive inadequacy.

♦ 6. This group usually lacks any real religious conviction.

♦ 7. This group is weak, easily controlled and take orders both at home and at their employment. They control no other adult in their lives.

♦ 8. This group harbors strong feelings of failure that are often realistic.

♦ 9. This group fears anger and avoids expressing anger themselves. They tend to be easy-going and need to be liked by everyone, especially children.

♦ 10. The major motivation of this group is seduction.

♦ 11. The victim for this group represents the offender in the past or an ideal self.

♦ 12. Victims can be of either sex and same-sex-sex is considered acceptable.

♦ 13. Sex must be enjoyable for the child more so than for himself. He needs to "please" the child.

INCESTUOUS FATHERS

♦ 1. These offenders have had successful adult sexual relationships and then regressed to below peer age levels.

♦ 2. This group is more adequate and are usually successful in most life situations.

♦ 3. This group frequently does quite well in employment. Many are successful business men or professionals.

♦ 4. This group has good relationships at work and socially outside the home. They are often considered model citizens.

♦ 5. These offenders are more socially skilled and display an excellent social facade.

♦ 6. This group is usually more religiously oriented, basically fundamentalists, but are hypocritical.

♦ 7. This group is characterized by the "King of the Castle Syndrome": They rule the lives of their wives and children and control all activities in and out of their homes.

♦ 8. Superiority often characterizes this group. Fears of failure, if they exist, are unrealistic.

♦ 9. This group is openly angry at their mothers and wives. Their anger ranges from mild to assaultive.

♦ 10. The major motivation of this group is anger.

♦ 11. The victim for this group represents his wife or girlfriend substitutes.

♦ 12. Victims are primarily females. Same-sex-sex is considered a "putdown," but boys are also victims.

♦ 13. Sexual behavior is to satisfy his own selfish, sexual pleasure. The sexual needs of the victim play no role.

Judy was a survivor and Donny was not. The depth of the effects on Donny are dramatically seen from one of his last journal entries:

☐ *"I wonder how it came to be that I was chosen to be the child of an animal— of a heartless bastard who comes from the pits of hell. I have spent my entire life in silent acceptance of what has had to be.— I never had an option or an alternative — there was no way that I could say no. Just grin and bear it.— No one would ever know what is at the core of my very sad soul— if in fact there is a soul left in me. It's full of crud."*

Donny took his own life, alone and in despair, on a hot balmy summer evening.

TREATMENT CONSIDERATIONS

In the past, even in our own treatment philosophy, it would have been considered essential to return to the original sexual trauma that determined the *victim-age-choice* and the *sexual-act-choice*. As this can be a long-term battle, especially where the original trauma is deeply repressed and defenses are formidable, we have since made this goal secondary to *immediate focus change*. The reasons are obvious:

- Since motivating the sex offender is an essential early treatment task, he must experience some immediate change or relief in order to believe that treatment can help. The constant problem of not remembering the trauma produces frustration and a belief that he is untreatable.

- It is a well-known axiom that with all clients in therapy, the harder you push and demand that a task (such as remembering) be accomplished, the less the chance of success.

- There are three essential requirements for change that must be met by the client:
    1. the *desire* to change;
    2. the *belief* that change is possible for me;
    3. the *belief* that I deserve to change.

We will discuss each of these requirements separately.

THE DESIRE TO CHANGE

Because clients come to therapists *stating* that they want to change, therapists often assume that this is true. Too often, this is not the truth. A very large number of clients that I have treated, eventually admitted to me in therapy that they really did not want to give up the deviant behavior. The reasons were myriad and included:

- "I really like what I'm doing and see nothing wrong with it!"
- "The kids like the sex and keep coming back for more, so it's not harming them. They know what they're doing!" (Pedophile/hebophile)
- "I've read a great deal and this behavior is not only normal in some societies but has been *proven* to help pre-adolescents grow and mature sexually." (Pedophile who is usually a NAMBLA member)
- "I know society says that what I'm doing is wrong but I disagree. It happened to me when I was a kid and never harmed me!" (Pedophile)
- "Women are always turning men on and then saying 'No'! How much do you think a man can take?" (Rapist)
- "She's/he's my kid and I can do anything I want to her/him." (Incest father)
- "He/she seduced me! All I did was respond to his/her seduction. What's wrong with that if it's his/her idea?" (Pedophile/hebophile)
- "My wife, kids, dog and car were all my possessions. That's how my father treated us and that's how I treat my family." (Incest father)
- "My rights take precedent over the whole family. After all I'm the breadwinner and without me they'd have nothing." (Incest father)

The resistance in these individuals, as well as their defensiveness, is extremely strong and rigid. Care must be taken not to be deceived by their initial protestations of sincerity, especially if the individual has been exposed and is now either facing court action or is already found guilty and is on probation with treatment as a condition.

As in many other treatment situations that will be discussed, *masturbation fantasies* will play an extremely important diagnostic role and thus need to be carefully monitored. Even fantasies that occur while the client is having sex with a partner are definite indicators of where the client is in his therapy. The claim that *"They (the deviant fantasies) keep coming back. I can't stop them!"* translates into: *"I keep using the fantasies to stimulate me and I don't really want* to give them up. I have a greater orgasm with my fantasies than with so-called normal ones."

Therapists must take special care not to allow the client to know what they are looking for. As stated in Chapter 1 and elsewhere, these are extremely clever and manipulative individuals who are "psyching" the therapist out as much as the therapist is trying to "psych" them out. An accepting, nonjudgmental approach, with homework assignments and self report, especially about fantasies, appears to be the best choice of technique.

Making absolutely sure that the client *wants to change* becomes a first hurdle and first priority. No further work can or will be accomplished until this desire to change is firmly established.

THE BELIEF THAT CHANGE IS POSSIBLE

Where change is concerned another often overlooked factor centers around the individual's own beliefs about his ability to change. While he may sincerely believe that change is possible for other deviates with identical symptoms and behaviors, it is quite possible for him to feel just as strongly that for him change is impossible. This then becomes a self- fulfilling prophesy.

Often there is a complex set of conscious or unconscious mechanisms functioning in this belief. For example: *if I really don't want to change or to give up my deviant behavior but cannot acknowledge or admit to this, what better way to accomplish my goal than to convince myself that change for me is impossible.* As opposed to the "desire to change" problems where supportive methods are employed to uncover the situation, here, *confrontation* may work better. This factor becomes readily visible in noncompliance to homework assignments with excuses such as "I forgot," or "I just didn't have time." When using confrontation methods, these alibis soon become *"I didn't want to!"* or *"What's the use, nothing works for me."*

As a general rule, *the longer the practice of the deviant behavior, the more likely that belief that change is impossible for him will remain a barrier to treatment.* In cases, where the child molester has had more than 100 victims and has been molesting for over 20 years, this factor emerges as the principal barrier to any real treatment progress and must become the principal focus of the therapy sessions.

Likewise, in the case of a rapist who has raped more than 60 women and successfully avoided arrest, this factor will present a serious barrier to all therapeutic efforts.

THE BELIEF THAT I DESERVE TO CHANGE

A simple sex offender formula explains:

- "If I change that will be positive; I will like myself more and people will also like me more. But I'm no good, bad, evil, etc., and I don't deserve all of these benefits. Therefore, I must not change."

In situations where the self-image and self-esteem are this poor, change is impossible until these negative judgments are modified to more positive ones. These are probably the most difficult cases to work with (even more difficult than the sociopaths). Formal therapy, as such, will produce few or no results. Insight, in my opinion and experience, does little to help and simply becomes an intellectual exercise for many in this specific group.

The only thing that appears to work consistently is to *set up situations and conditions where the client will be forced to succeed and also be unable to deny the success.* I have used art work, sports, home improvement and repair, electronics and many other related daily activities to *prove* to the client that he is worth something. Beginning with *physical* forms of success, I then move to *social* and *moral* forms of success. For example, helping a friend or neighbor, saying "no!" just once to an impulse, substituting a good behavior for a bad one, etc. Each success is recorded and a record (list) kept of each successful incident and the *worth* attached to it. The following simple logic becomes an important aide: *Could an evil, worthless, no good person do all of these highly positive things?*

The first and most desired effect is for the client to begin having doubts about his worthlessness and then slowly to begin to believe that, *possibly*, he is worth something. This slow change method works better than any fast and dramatic seeming improvement, and is more credible with the client.

THERAPIST CAUTIONS

When dealing with sex offenders, either institutionalized or in the community, whether self-referred or on probation, therapists have a moral and ethical responsibility to the community and the potential victims that these individuals could harm. It is quite easy for the offender to *rationalize* that as long as he is coming to therapy, he is being treated. This is not always true!

In Chapter 10, we discussed the need for *confirmation* to be the method of choice with these individuals. Several additional factors will be considered at this point.

A time limit should be established for evaluating discernible change and/or other indicators of therapeutic progress.

Dennis attended weekly therapy sessions with no visible or reported change in over six months. When I asked him why he continued coming and spending his money, he replied *"Because I need treatment, I'm a sick person."*

Then I asked if he thought he was receiving treatment, and he stated *"Of course I am, you're a therapist, aren't you?"* I then set immediate limits for some positive effort and results and gave him a month to begin making some movement towards change. Surprisingly, he did improve on a social and interpersonal level but *refused to give up his deviant masturbation practices and fantasies* stating, *"There's no way I can stop doing it now. That will take a long, long time for me to stop, if ever."*

Each step of the way in treatment with this type of individual is a battle for both control and change. Each therapist must make up his/her own mind as to how long he/she can be the *excuse and alibi* for an offender who is still free in the community.

Therapists working with offenders in the community must realize that treatment strips away defense mechanisms and that the client will, in all likelihood, get worse before he gets better.

This principle also applies pointedly to Dennis. When he began treatment, his masturbation fantasies involved seven- or eight-year-old boys with only their shirts off standing across the room from his bed. He then fantasized an older boy punching them in the stomach and that brought him to his climax. As therapy progressed, the fantasies *changed* and frightened both the client and the therapist: In the new fantasy, the boy was now totally nude and the fantasy was of Dennis walking over to him and fondling him. Without the change, Dennis could no longer reach a climax. The dangers are obvious.

The therapist must constantly re-evaluate each case as to progress, potential danger to himself or others and the ability of the offender to remain safely in the community.

There will come a time in many of these cases where the fuse is lit and the danger to the community becomes too great for the therapist to continue with the same treatment. What then? Options depend on the circumstances.

- If the client is on probation, that department should be informed of the therapist's concerns *without divulging any confidential material*. There is usually a condition that the therapist must provide regular evaluations on the progress or lack of progress of the probationer. After several frightening cases of this type in my early years of treating offenders, I made it a condition, when I received a referral from the courts, that regular evaluations and progress reports would be required and that the court or probation department would arrange for the legal releases of such reports. Since that decision, I have had little trouble with these cases.

- In cases where the client is self-referred and not on probation, the problem is a little more complicated but can still be dealt with. Once adequate rapport is established and the client trusts the therapist, he/she usually will accept the advice that is given. On several occasions I was forced to recommend inpatient treatment at a private facility when the overt dangers to the community became too great. This decision relieved the burden as well as the anxiety of both the client and the therapist.

Once a sex offender, whether he is currently committing offenses or not, is removed from the specific source of his temptations there is a relief that nothing else can provide, a feeling of being *safe*.

Finally, in cases of parolees, the problem becomes simpler. Referrals from the parole department automatically involve updates and evaluative reports on a regular basis. Additionally, the parole officers usually have the right to detain and rearrest offenders who behave in a manner that suggests an *imminent danger of return to their criminal behavior or a threat to the community.* The need to become involved in any of the above situations should remain a major consideration before a therapist decides to specialize in this controversial and responsibility-laden area.

13

Rapists Versus Seductive Offenders

In 1962, having just completed an internship at a state reformatory for boys, I transferred to the now-defunct New Jersey State Diagnostic Center as a first level, wet-behind- the-ears psychologist. I had dealt with several cases of sexual offenses, both offenders and victims, at the reformatory during my internship, and my interest was now fairly well-established.

The very first case I was assigned to involved rape. That was all I was told. I would be a member of a three-person team (psychiatrist, psychologist, and psychiatric social worker) who would have 90 days to evaluate the case and send a recommendation to the courts as to how the offender should be handled. Our choices were:

- return him/her to their home on strict probation with outpatient treatment,
- incarcerate him/her at a state reformatory or
- send him/her to a residential treatment center for a specified period of time.

The case involved a rapist who had assaulted three young girls in a grammar school. A knock on my office door began my real education into the world of sexual pathology.

☐ *In walked* SKIPPY, *a three-foot six-inch, 40 to 45 pound, skinny and openly assertive seven year old boy. At this point, I was sure that this was my initiation by the staff. Nothing could be further from the truth. Skippy had been arrested for the rape of three of his female schoolmates. In addition, he smoked at least a full pack of cigarettes a day and could not sleep without drinking a six pack of beer. All of these facts were verified in his folder by the investigating juvenile detective.*

From this first visit and for several more to come, a confrontational relationship developed between Skippy and me. He was not the least bit inhibited and had an adult sexual vocabulary (slang). Rather than being frightened or embarrassed by his situation, as most other children his age were at the Center, Skippy took pride in his "macho" (his word) accomplishments. He intimidated the other children on his housing wing and even some of the staff. Whenever he got angry at me for pushing too hard in an area he did not want to discuss, he threatened to urinate on me.

How could this have happened? The literature available in 1962 was of little help and it became quickly apparent that only Skippy knew the answers to the puzzle! Through many, many hours of establishing rapport and trust with Skippy — we eventually became good friends — the following facts emerged.

☐ *Skippy and his mother came to the United States from Puerto Rico looking for streets lined with gold. They had lived in abject poverty in Puerto Rico and felt their only hope was to come to the United States. They settled in a largely Hispanic city that was known in New Jersey as "Little Puerto Rico." Skippy's mother soon discovered that there was little work for her since she spoke practically no English and had no skills. Friends found a single room for her and her young son in a rooming house and, rather than starve or return to Puerto Rico, Skippy's mother made a living the only way she knew how: she prostituted.*

At this time, Skippy was between two and three years old (as far as investigators could determine) and, since there was no money for a babysitter, he sat or lay on the bed while his mother serviced her customers. Eventually, Skippy admitted that some of the customers preferred him to his mother and, as a result, he was molested on a regular basis. After a period of time, he felt like this was normal behavior and admitted that, at times, he enjoyed the sex as well as the gifts and affection the male customers lavished on him. His poor mother told him how proud she was of her "real man" since Skippy's father deserted them when he found out that the mother was pregnant. They had never been married and so she had no legal recourse.

The real trauma occurred when Skippy was six- years- old and was sent out to school. Innocently, he told his newly found friends (boys and girls alike) about his mother's "friends" and the games they all played. He was immediately ostracized by both the children and the teachers. Their comments were hurtful and insulting and, for the first time in his life, Skippy learned to hate. From that point on, Skippy became a serious behavioral problem: fighting, stealing, smoking and drinking beer. Vandalism became an outlet, especially where female teachers were concerned.

At no time, did Skippy tell his mother what was happening at school and they both continued earning their subsistence through sex. By early age seven he had heard about fags and queers and his anger turned into uncontrollable rage. He began to daydream about showing everyone that he was "macho" and not a "chulo" (a male-prostitute). Being too small to attempt an assault on an adult woman (the fantasies centered about one specific sadistic female teacher at school), he chose schoolmates who rejected him and made fun of his speech, clothing, and his difficulty in learning to read. The rapes resulted.

WHY RAPE?

Skippy's anger and rage, while consciously directed at the sadistic teacher and then projected onto his age mates, was, on a deeper level, directed at his mother. After many, many therapy sessions that were always emotional, threatening and quite stormy, Skippy was finally willing to explore the possibility that he was really angry at his mother. He was asked to *imagine* possible reasons that he might have for being angry with his mother and the following emerged:

- She was poor.
- She did not have a husband and therefore Skippy did not have a father.
- She earned a living through prostitution.
- She could not speak English well and this embarrassed him.
- She was not getting him out of the Center.

Finally, after many difficult sessions came the real key to the anger:

- She allowed the men to *use him* homosexually and he was still fantasizing to those homosexual acts and even masturbating to them.

This last reason was paramount, since Skippy felt that it made him a *"queer"* or *"fag"* and he had to deny it. In many of the rape cases we have seen and treated, regardless of the fact that a male was the molester during the rapist's youth, the *mother* was the one he deeply blamed. Developmentally, children see the mother as their *protector*, not the father or father-figure. Therefore, regardless of who sexually traumatized the rapist as a child or adolescent, he sees it as the mother's fault for not protecting him by knowing what was happening and preventing it.

The rapist tends to develop an *extreme dependence* on his mother that prevents him from venting any rage he feels directly on her. Instead he *displaces* the rage on a substitute female who either in looks, behavior or attitude reminds him of his mother and thus triggers the rage to the surface. The victim could also be someone that the mother appears (in the distorted mind of the rapist) to love more than him. Thus the substitute victim could be *anyone*: a student, a neighbor, an employee, or even a total stranger. Note, however, that in child molesters, the anger would most likely be aimed at the mother's favorite: his brother or sister or even one of his friends.

REPRESSION

JOEY, now an adult rapist, came from a family of marital conflicts. When Joey was around 12-years-old, the following set of circumstances occurred:

☐ *Joey's father began to take him out every Saturday, explaining to Joey's mother that he and his son needed more time alone to become friends and to get to know each other better since Joey was entering adolescence. Joey's mother believed the story. In reality, Joey's father was using him as an alibi to visit his secret paramour. Joey would be given a game or some comic books to read and instructed to sit on the porch of the paramour's home while the father visited upstairs.*

Joey was quite street-wise by age 12 and knew or fantasized what he felt was going on upstairs. However, as long as his father treated him well, bought him gifts and later took him somewhere such as an amusement park, swimming pool or bowling alley, he really didn't care. He also wanted and needed the individual attention he was getting from his father and was unwilling to upset the applecart.

These Saturday excursions continued for more than six months until a dramatic change occurred. One day, as he was reading a comic book on the front porch of the paramour's home, his father came down in his underwear and took Joey by the hand, leading him upstairs. Upon entering the bedroom, the frightened Joey became aware of two things: (1) a naked woman, quite large, lying on a frilly bed, and (2) a strong odor of cheap perfume. Joey's father ordered him to undress and when he hesitated, the father undressed him, stating, "It's about time you became a man, if you're good enough!" The boy was then ordered to lie on top of the woman and to "show me what kind of a man you are!"

Though he knew about sexual intercourse, Joey was a virgin and, under the circumstances, was so frightened and confused that he could not get an erection. The woman (he never was told her name) put her arms around him, held him tightly and whispered in his ear, "Be a good boy, Joey, and don't cry."

Joey, more frightened and confused than ever, felt his father climbing on top of him. The next thing he felt was terrible anal pain as his father penetrated him. Joey now was in shock and the woman kept trying to calm and comfort him. When the father was finally finished, he said: "Boy, you've got the best and tightest 'pussy' I've ever had!"

Joey was never to forget this phrase, which to him meant that his father had used him as a woman. When they left the house, not a word was spoken between them. Upon arriving home, Joey was obviously in pain and wet since he was bleeding quite a bit. His mother treated his bleeding by packing cotton up his rectum (a second rape). She never asked a single question as to what happened and Joey assumed that she knew what his father had done to him and really didn't care.

From this point on, Joey became a real behavior problem both at home and in school. He was constantly disrespectful to his teachers and to his mother, and was always getting into fights and doing all sorts of daring feats to prove his strength and his masculinity. In less than a full year after that episode, Joey committed his first rape on a high school girl that he so terrified and threatened that she never reported it. Joey was on his way to becoming a compulsive rapist and by the time he was finally apprehended, some eight years later, he had raped more than 25 women.

During his first year or more of therapy, there was no conscious memory of his own rape. Joey had *repressed* the entire incident. He had rationalized his rapes on his difficulties in all female relationships and the resulting anger and rage he felt at being ridiculed, rejected or putdown by females, regardless of age.

Before we continue, an explanation of repression may be necessary. Repression can be best understood in the following definition (Wolman, 1989, p. 292):

Repression is an unconscious exclusion from the consciousness of objectionable impulses, memories, and ideas. The ego, as it were, pushes the objectionable material down into the unconscious and acts as if the objectionable material were nonexistent.

Thus, one of the most difficult problems faced in treating these individuals, as well as their victims (survivors), is to discover whether there are any repressions and, if there are repressions suspected, to bring them to the conscious level. The following rule or guideline may be helpful in determining whether or not a repression exists in a particular case: *Whenever a compulsive behavior is discovered that has no logical explanation or etiology, look for a repressed trauma.* This is especially true where *compulsive ritual* is concerned. Several examples of such rituals may shed some light on the concept.

Choosing a Particular Setting

☐ *Skippy always lured his potential victims to his room and assaulted them in his mother's bed. (By this time, his mother had found employment and was no longer prostituting.)*

☐ *Joey always broke into apartments or homes and assaulted women in their own bedroom. If this was not possible, then he would take them to a "cheap and crummy hotel since that was all that whores deserved."*

☐ *Kevin consistently used the backyards of homes where he had been stalking his victims.*

Finding Victims in a Particular Place

☐ *Skippy's victims were always classmates from school.*

☐ *Joey always chose women in diners or bars, nowhere else.*

☐ *Kevin always cruised middle-class neighborhoods and chose women who were out late at night, walking home alone.*

Looking for Victims Exhibiting a Specific Behavior Pattern

☐ *Skippy's victims always had to be female classmates who directly or indirectly put him down or made him feel below them.*

☐ *Joey always chose women who were seductive and came on to him.*

☐ *Kevin always chose women who appeared weak and defenseless and who also appeared pious and proper.*

Following Certain Set(s) of Behaviors During the Assault

☐ *Skippy always made the girls undress and lie naked on the bed (as he remembered his mother doing) and then smile and act astonished at his erect penis size.*

☐ *Joey always made his victims kneel, beg, ask permission to fellate him, take his pants down and after he was aroused beg him to rape them. They also had to tell him that his performance was great after he climaxed. (All of this was accomplished by threat and a knife).*

☐ *Kevin always forced his victims to choose between fellating him or being raped. He preferred the fellatio but would do whatever they chose.*

RAPE AS OVERCOMPENSATION FOR PERCEIVED MALE SEXUAL INADEQUACY

One of the most frequent underlying dynamics of rape is *an overwhelming (compulsive) need to prove masculinity*. These individuals, for reasons that only they know, lack feelings of masculinity in their sexual performance as well as in many or all other aspects of their lives. Reality has little to do with these feelings, as often the significant- others in their lives feel the opposite is true. Their daily appearance and behavior also often contradict the perceived deficiency. An example will clarify:

☐ TED, *from his earliest memories, was raised in a totally female environment. He never knew his father and, to this day, has no idea of who his father was or why the man abandoned him. The women in his home included his mother, his grandmother and two spinster aunts, who all hated men with a vengeance. As a consequence of this misanthropic situation, each time Ted arrived home from anywhere (going to the store, playing in the yard alone, visiting a friend, returning from school), he was made to undress completely in the foyer of the house and then to re- dress from the skin outwards into female clothing. In the house, he was called* TEDDY *but in a manner which intimated that he was a girl, not a boy. His chores were traditionally female tasks; he was taught skills and crafts such as needlepoint, cooking and housekeeping tasks and was never allowed to play typical boys's games. Even his toilet behavior was feminine, as he was made to sit down to urinate and to be sure his penis was never seen or touched. Through this conditioning, his mannerisms became totally feminine and he was labeled a sissy by the neighbors as well as his teachers and peers when he began school. The fact that he was good-looking, in a soft way, added to the problem.*

At adolescence, Ted did not develop physically and at age 16 he still had the body and genitals of an 11-year- old pre-pubescent boy. The teasing in high school was intense and Ted began acting out in passive-aggressive ways, such as stealing other pupil's belongings (especially those who taunted him) or hiding to avoid gym classes. Eventually his anger and rage burst into vandalism. Once he came to the attention of the juvenile justice system, he was removed from his environment and placed in a foster home. He was physically examined and given hormone shots to induce adolescence. (Interestingly, the physician could never find a physical cause for the lack of pubertal development and concluded that somehow it was all psychologically based.) He began to grow physically and to develop sexually, and quickly learned all the myths about sex from other boys in the home.

Ted's first dating attempt at his high school prom was a disaster. He was awkward, could not dance and stammered badly when he tried to communicate. He felt an anger in the company of his date that he did not understand. He tolerated the situation for as long as he could and then disappeared from the prom, abandoning his date. The ridicule and censure he received at school the next Monday was too much and he ran away. While hitchhiking, he was picked up by an older woman who attempted to seduce him by rubbing his leg and crotch. Again he felt the rage and panicked, jumping out of the moving car and hiding in the woods where he fell asleep. He awoke to the singing of a 16- year-old girl walking home from church, and without even thinking, jumped from the woods, grabbed her and dragged her into the shrubbery where he raped her under threat of her life.

Ted was arrested walking down the same road within an hour of the rape and was sent to the treatment unit. Prison terrified him, and living in a large open dormitory with open bathrooms and showers was even more terrifying. However, contrary to his expectations, the men in the unit adopted him as a sort of mascot or younger brother whom they protected and advised. In therapy, Ted was totally open (again due to his immaturity and naivete) and painfully verbalized what had been done to him in childhood and the lingering effects of feeling feminine. He also stated that he felt that he should have been born a girl.

While psychotherapy dealt with his conditioning, his anger and his self-image problems on one level, the group members took on the task of "masculinizing" Ted. They taught him sports on a basic level, taught him to play pool, workout in the gym (after a year of therapy) and lower his voice to sound more manly. As his therapist, I encouraged him to release his anger *as it occurred* if it were appropriate (certainly not with the prison officers). He did so in therapy situations or with his peers in the dormitory.

In three years, while the feminine traits were still visible from time to time (especially when he was embarrassed and blushed from ear to ear), Ted appeared to be a new person who acted masculine for the most part and much more openly assertive than ever before.

Six months after his release he met a hometown girl and married her. They have three children and, at his last check- in, were doing quite well. What was done to Ted was not an active sexual molestation but was definitely a passive sexual trauma for him. Other forms of *identity conflicts* that may also result in sexually deviant behavior are described below.

The "You Are A Failure!" Cases

☐ *Dennis, whom we met in Chapter 6, comes from an old- world family with a passive-compliant mother and a dominant, tyrannical father whose word is law. Dennis' older brother was the favorite of both parents, and Dennis was told by his parents early in his childhood that he was an "unexpected gift from God that made life difficult for the whole family."*

From this point onward, his life was full of misery and rejection. No matter what he did, it was never good enough and the father's persistent prediction was that Dennis would never amount to anything. Desperate for acceptance, Dennis tried even harder, and the harder he tried the more often he failed in his father's eyes. Looking to his mother or his older brother for support was a waste of time and Dennis soon learned to stop trying. This became the pattern for his whole life: at home, in school and playing with other children (a rare occurrence since most of the time he was an observer).

Somehow, he squeaked into college and eventually graduated with a C average. His parents were unimpressed, and did not even have a party or celebration for his graduation. Dennis found a menial job in his chosen field (television broadcasting), but here again he isolated, never socialized with other employees after work and never really tried for promotion. When, at age 29, he began to take an inordinate interest in six to seven-year-old boys, he requested therapy.

Throughout his therapeutic involvement of over one full year, he has made only minimal progress in any area. He begins each session by enumerating the *failures* of the previous week, looking for the rebuke and punishment he would receive from his father (this factor is now conscious and accepted). Both Dennis and the therapist remain frustrated at his lack of real growth. Recently, Dennis finally stated: *"I guess I'm so used to being a failure that I'm comfortable this way and know how to act. If I change, I'll have to try new things and that is too frightening. I guess I'll stay this way."*

While this certainly is his right, the problem is that his attraction for young boys has become overtly sexual and he is masturbating to fantasies of fondling them. If some therapeutic intervention is not found soon, another victim of child sexual abuse will soon exist.

The "Who Am I?" Cases

The following case exemplifies the "Who Am I?" case quite lucidly.

☐ LARRY *was a handsome, well-built, athletic instructor for a local health club. He was in college and hoped to become either a teacher of physical education or possibly a lawyer. Although his father had deserted the family when Larry was only nine or ten, he seemed to have found sufficient male figure substitutes to develop along normal lines. He was the most popular male in his senior high school class, and was elected class president and voted most likely to succeed. Larry's mother was a hard-working domestic for a wealthy family who wanted only the best for her son, and tried to be both mother and father. One day, Larry was searching for his high school diploma and went through his mother's private papers. To his total shock he found his birth certificate and learned that he was illegitimate, and that his father was a well-known millionaire, living in the same town but in a much different neighborhood.*

Feelings of anger, rage, hatred, confusion and depression all fused and he went out and got sickeningly drunk. When he came home, he confronted his mother and she told him the whole story. She had worked for the father's family, and became pregnant. However, she did not fit in the family's plans for their son, so they gave her a small amount of hush-money and paid her medical bills for the pregnancy. She had had no contact with his father since and to her knowledge he had never seen or known his own son nor did he want to.

Larry attempted to see his father but was refused admittance to the mansion and told that it was impossible for him to be related to this great man. While consciously feeling anger and hatred for his father, Larry began mistreating women at the health club where he worked and was terse and defiant towards his mother. Within five months, he was picking up prostitutes and having violent sex with them attempting to make it as painful as possible and then literally throwing them out of his car without paying for their services. On the third or fourth such incident, the prostitute hollered rape and Larry was given a 30 year sentence to the treatment unit. Therapy was quite rapid since he was open and quickly revealed the real problem, his illegitimacy, and the meaning he put on it: "I'm inferior, dirty, useless, unwanted," and/or "I don't deserve having clean and good girls, only prostitutes who are as bad as . . . . . .???" Eventually the ending became: "My mother!"

In 18 months, Larry was released and returned to both his job with the hotel chain and to college. Today he is a successful attorney (this required special exemption from the morals code of the Bar which a state senator helped him to gain). Larry is married and has two boys of his own who are helping him to regain the missing father-son childhood he was deprived of. The terribly sad thing about both of these cases is that had they been discovered early enough and treated appropriately, the sexually deviant behavior (in both cases: rape) could have been avoided. This is where communication between parents and children, as well as sex education in the home and in the school, with peer discussion included, could make all of the difference in these children's lives.

14

The Sex Offender's Motivation May Not Be Sexual

In all my years of dealing with sex offenders, both in a correctional setting (convicted and sentenced) and in private practice (referred, self referred or on probation), *I have never encountered a case where* sex was the primary motivation. In all of the cases I have treated or examined, one or a combination of the following primary motivations could easily be identified:

- *Power/domination* needs (in all sexual assaults and incest)
- *Seductive/acceptance* needs (in all child molestation)
- *Ritual/undoing* needs (in either sexual assault or child molestation)

POWER /DOMINATION NEEDS

Two major groups of offenders will be found with power and/or domination needs: the sexually assaultive personalities (rapists, assaultive child molesters, etc.) and the incest fathers group. Where sexual assault is concerned, the power/domination elements are clearly visible and understood. These individuals come under the *deny-ers* category (see Chapter 2). They are grossly overcompensating for their perceived inadequacies.

Sexual assault ranges from minimal to sadistic and is a *progressive* pathology in that these individuals tend to increase the force, anger and injuries to the victim until the ultimate sexual assault is reached, i.e., *murder*. Having control over the life of the victim gives the offender *power*, a desperate need, since for the majority of their lives they have felt powerless.

The sexual component is not uniform in this group. Not all sexually assaultive persons commit rape (vaginal penetration) or sodomy (anal penetration). For some, depending on their own original sexual trauma, oral sex (one-sided or mutual) is the act of choice; for others, a variety of deviant acts may be forced upon the victim including analingus, urophilia, and even coprophilia.

At this point, let us consider three ascending degrees of sexual assault.

In **Stage 1 assaults,** the distinguishing characteristics are these:

- Minimal physical force is used in the offense. The sexually assaultive person primarily uses threat, coercion, physical overpowering and may show but not use a weapon to achieve his end.

- Abusive and degrading language is used and may include cursing, demeaning insults, accusations and obscene putdowns.

- The victim is often forced to say that she/he enjoyed the act or that she/he loves the offender. The purpose here is to assuage the resulting guilt of the offender which occurs as soon as he reaches orgasm, and also to justify his behavior.

- Once the sexual act is completed, this group tends to become guilt ridden and even remorseful. They have been known to attempt to comfort their victims and even to drive them to their homes or to a hospital. (Many have been captured doing just this!)

- The assaults tend to occur following a sudden *trigger,* and are not premeditated. Any occurrence that triggers the sexually assaultive person's feelings of being controlled, being put down or being rejected can trigger an attack.

- Rather than following a ritual, the assaults can take place anywhere, anytime and in any manner.

In **Stage 2 sexual assaults,** the distinguishing characteristics are:

- The sexually assaultive person uses as much force as he feels is necessary to subjugate the victim and to accomplish his goals of both complete control and sexual submission to his most deviant fantasies.

• Control and threat are the main themes of his language. He repeatedly verbalizes his control to the victim and poses the possible dangers that she/he faces unless there is a total conformity to his will.

• The sexually assaultive person usually demands *silence* on the part of the victim and often orders the victim to either close her/his eyes or not to look at him or what he is doing. A blindfold is frequently used.

• Physical harm to the victim is frequent and includes bloody noses, sprained arms, facial battering and even minor cutting with a knife *"just to prove who is in control and what can happen if you don't do exactly what I want!"* The physical harm and injury are primarily a result of his seething rage (over which he has lost control) and secondly due to his need to punish the victim for what someone else has done to him. This rage usually results from his own sexual molestation and/or trauma.

• The assaults are more premeditated and planned than those in Stage 1. The offender becomes obsessed with thoughts of revenge and anger (to the point of uncontrolled rage) and masturbates compulsively to rape and assault fantasies. The assault is usually the outcome of his fantasies being perpetrated on a victim in reality, when he no longer can maintain control.

• When the assault is over, the offender cares little for the victim and often leaves her/him where the attack occurred, giving strict orders for her/him not to move or cry out for help for a period of time. There is also the extended threat that if she/he goes to the authorities or tries to identify him that he *"knows who she/he is and where she/he lives and he will come back and get her/him!"*

In **Stage 3 sexual assaults**, the principal features are:

• Force is *sadistically* employed to ventilate anger and rage, not because the victim is unwilling to cooperate. The sadism includes cutting, burning and various other forms of torture. Bondage is employed as a control method and to ensure that the victim does not fight back. It is not uncommon for the offender to bludgeon the victim into unconsciousness and then undress and tie the victim up, often in her/his own bed.

• The sex acts are made painful, degrading and humiliating. In intercourse, the offender uses his penis like a *battering ram*, deliberately causing pain for the victim even if he experiences pain himself. He may make the victim lick his penis clean (see Harry, Chapter 5, pp. 48-49) or perform analingus just to add to the humiliation and degradation.

- If the offender suspects the victim is enjoying the sex, he will become furious and change the act or make sure that he inflicts pain to the point of bleeding or physical damage.

- Power and anger needs dominate the entire experience and the offender will do anything necessary to prove to the victim that he is in complete control of the victim's life.

- The assaults may take place over an extended period of time. Often the victim has been kidnapped and taken to a safe and isolated area where the sexually assaultive person can keep the victim for his own use as long as he wants, even for weeks at a time.

- The sexually assaultive person tends to *panic* and fear capture and punishment, after he finishes and empties his vast need for revenge and retaliation (displaced from his own life experiences onto the victim). This is the most dangerous part of the assault for the victim and, not infrequently, results in the victim's death.

The above three degrees of sexual assault are not intended to be all-encompassing. There are as many varieties of sexual assault as there are individuals perpetrating these assaults. Each sexually assaultive person is an individual with unique needs and his own deviant practices. Each time I felt that I had seen the final type of assault, I met a new offender with a new set of needs and methods of satisfying them.

SEDUCTION/ACCEPTANCE NEEDS

Three groups of offenders will be found with these needs: the seductive pedophiles, the seductive hebophiles and the seductive incest fathers. The term *seductive* is a necessary prefix to each of these groups since there are also parallel *assaultive* types of pedophiles, hebophiles and incest fathers.

These groups are composed of the *most inadequate* of all of the sex offenders. They are frightened of and repulsed by any form of violence, no matter how minimal. Some of their traits include:

- Their overall desperate need is for *acceptance* from their victims.

- They are gentle, friendly, kind and persuasive.

- They use money, gifts, special privileges, friendship and other seductions to accomplish their goals.

- Their patience is incredible and rather than surrender to their sexual needs, they take care to first form a trusting and caring relationship with the intended victim.
- The goal of their initial sexual exploration with the victim is to *please and satisfy* them so that the victim will not only like him but also so that they will *return for more.*
- Their choice of sex act is totally dependent on their own early sexual molestation and/or sexual trauma.
- They are manipulative, cunning, seductive and prefer to *psych-out* their victims rather than use force of any kind. The one exception is their tendency to use photographs as a form of *blackmail.*

The pedophile and hebophile groups have large numbers of different victims. I have had offenders with as many as 600 verified cases. These large numbers of victims are due to the fact that even *successful* molestations *do not meet the offender's needs!* They are never satisfied with the acceptance and love they feel they are receiving from their present victim *but they can't explain why.* They continue to look for one victim after another. Each time they fantasize that "this will be the one I've been looking for!" — but it never works.

The issue of course, is simple to state but very difficult to treat: *The real need is for love and acceptance from the parent of their childhood, at the time where the trauma occurred and the need was generated.* Even admitting this insight to themselves can take years of therapy and confrontation. Communicating this insight to their parent (if she/he is still alive) is an even more formidable task. However, without this admission, the problem will never be fully resolved.

RITUAL UNDOING NEEDS

Ritual undoing is a defense reaction of many sexually abused children who never reported or resolved their trauma through some form of therapy. In these cases the offenders, often as adolescents or young adults, find a victim who is of the same age, general appearance and personality-type that they were at the time they were abused and *repeat the sexual abuse in the exact same manner* that occurred during their own abuse. This often includes the same setting, the same seduction or threat, the same acts, etc. In this way, they hope to *undo* or *normalize* what happened to them.

An example will clarify:

☐ LEON *was raped at the age of 12 in a state reformatory where he had been sent for school truancy. At the time, he was small of build, shy, timid and unable to defend himself. Additionally, he was quite a good-looking young boy and friendly to all (a mistake in a reformatory). He trusted an older youth who was the duke (leader and strongest boy of the cottage who is trusted by the cottage parents to be left in charge while they are away).*

After an initial period of friendliness and protection, the duke decided it was time for Leon to pay for his friendship. One night, he assigned Leon to mop the downstairs shower room after lights out and while Leon was doing his chores, the duke came down and forcibly raped him. From that day on, Leon trusted no one and his self-worth (what little he had) was destroyed. When released from the reformatory, Leon could not readjust to society. He was always in trouble, hated and resented anyone in authority over him and began flashing. At age 22, he was caught and sent to the sex offender treatment unit where I met him. He worked as a clerk in the office, was a well-behaved and well-liked inmate and never received a disciplinary report. One morning, he declared an emergency and I interviewed him in my office. He painfully and tearfully confessed to raping one of the new, younger, shy, and frightened inmates, whom he perceived as being similar to himself at 12 in the reformatory. When I asked him why he had committed the rape, he stated: "Now I'm not the only one!"

However, within a week, Leon returned to say that his undoing did not last and that the old negative feelings of being dirty, used and unworthy had all returned. He was feeling intense guilt for what he had done to the younger inmate who had trusted him. I suggested that he bring the problem to his primary group and he did. The group, while shocked and angry, did not reject Leon or ask for his removal from the group. Instead they asked how they could help and all rallied around him. They also suggested that he now help the young inmate he raped to deal with his feelings and reactions to the sexual assault. To aid this process, I transferred the new victim from another group to Leon's primary group. From that day on, Leon's progress in therapy accelerated; he became a group leader and worked hard and diligently with the young male he raped. In helping his victim to realize that it was not his fault, that it didn't make him a bad person or dirty etc., he began to accept the same messages for himself. Within a month, Leon's demeanor began to change and he became more assertive, more open with criticism and positive feedback in group and earned the respect of everyone in the treatment unit. In a year or so he was released. Nine months later, he married and has been doing well without a recurrence for the last ten or more years.

If it were possible for all sex offenders to work in the same group with their victims, therapy could be accelerated and be much more positive in its outcome. However, this is not always a practical or workable solution and other means must be found to alter the negative self-image.

THE DANGER OF SYMPTOM SUBSTITUTION

One of the most serious mistakes that was made during my first year of dealing with sex offenders was overlooking the dangers of *symptom substitution.* One of our therapists was an expert in behavior modification techniques. At that time, none of us really knew how to treat offenders and so we each tried our own expertise first and then discussed results.

☐ KEN, *a 31-year-old rapist whom we met in Chapter 6, admitted readily to at least three other rapes although this was his first arrest and conviction. Ken was an extremely bright (WAIS I.Q. 140+), well-educated young man with a smooth social approach to everyone. He came from a fairly wealthy family (country club, flower club, politics, etc.) that was totally supportive (especially his mother and sister) throughout his treatment and institutionalization. From day one, Ken was open and revealing in group and soon became his group's leader and spokesman. He utilized very few recognizable defense mechanisms and made very rapid progress. Ken's behavior was exemplary and he soon earned a high position of trust in the prison (Captain's clerk) and was respected by inmates and staff alike.*

After 18 months in the treatment unit he was paroled. While initial readjustment appeared excellent, he was never perceived as being happy.

As we discussed in Chapter 6, after visiting me in the hospital to ask for a recommendation to graduate school, Ken committed another rape.

Driving out of the parking lot, he followed another visitor (a young, attractive girl) to the garages in the rear of her apartment complex, overpowered and raped her and then walked away directly towards the police station, a half-mile away, where he was apprehended. Ken was returned to the treatment center and then admitted that he had lied in therapy and withheld important factors such as his rage and anger at a wealthy relative whom he perceived as mistreating his mother.

As was our practice, Ken should have been reassigned to his old therapist (me!). It was apparent that I had been fooled the first time and that it would be wise to assign Ken to another therapist. His new therapist was a specialist in behavior modification techniques, and Ken again was treated basically in this modality. After four years, he was released for the second time on parole. Within a year of release Ken was rearrested on a charge of conspiracy to murder the above mentioned relative and is serving a life sentence for that offense. Fortunately I was able to interview him for a lengthy time and the gist of what he told me was that the sexual aspects of the therapy worked well. He never wanted to rape again and his sex life with his fiancee was excellent. As you will see however, we had been conned again.

Ken never let go of or resolved the rage he felt for the relative whom he felt was abusing his mother. His displaced anger towards women still existed, but now the outlet was physical, not sexual. Working exclusively on the symptom simply converted the symptom into another outlet and the plans to kill the offending relative resulted.

In our experience, behavior modification *alone,* as with any other treatment technique with offenders used alone, in our experience, does not seem to work. This was especially true where anger and rage were concerned. *A confrontational approach, aimed at the release of any and all emotion, remains, in our experience, an effective treatment choice when utilized with ancillary programs to deal with other aspects of the offender's personality makeup.*

MASTURBATORY RECONDITIONING

There is a particular type of sex offender who, no matter how hard he works in therapy and no matter how much intellectual insight he develops, is unable to eradicate his obsessions with his own form of sexual deviation. These obsessive fantasies and daydreams are especially persistent when he is alone with nothing to do. They result in masturbation to the deviant fantasy, *no matter how hard he tries to avoid it and no matter what promises he makes to himself each time it occurs.* The consistent result is guilt that prevents self-esteem from improving and a resistant judgment that he will never be able to change or get better.

DENNIS (whom we met in Chapters 6, 12 and 13) has had such a masturbatory problem for over ten years and uses it to destroy any progress he makes, due to a still undiscovered trauma that fuels the guilt. Regardless of how well he does at work or in a social situation, at night, after fighting and resisting for hours and hours, always ends up with the same deviant masturbation fantasy. He has convinced himself that he will never be able to achieve orgasm without his deviant fantasy of little boys.

One of the techniques that I have found successful in dealing with this type of unwanted, undesirable, deviant masturbatory fantasy problem is a modified form of masturbatory reconditioning. There are several types of reconditioning to be found in the literature including a form called *satiation,* which I found over the years does not work well in my practice with compulsive sex offenders. As early as 1969, I modified the then-known techniques and developed my own form.

MASTURBATORY RECONDITIONING TECHNIQUE

For compulsive masturbation to deviant fantasies followed by guilt, instruct the client to follow these eight steps *exactly:*

- 1. When you find yourself masturbating to a deviant fantasy, allow it to continue up to the p.e.i. (pre- ejaculatory inevitability) phase.
- 2. Never allow orgasm to be reached using the deviant fantasy.
- 3. Have a positive fantasy prepared (in writing) to use when the p.e.i. phase is reached. This fantasy should be pre-approved by a therapist.
- 4. When *p.e.i.* is reached, switch the deviant fantasy to the positive fantasy and reach orgasm and ejaculation.
- 5. Do the exercise *no fewer than three times a week for at least two weeks to one month, and always* when the deviant fantasy occurs.
- 6. Following orgasm, *evaluate* why the masturbation to the deviant fantasy occurred; in particular, focus on identifying the *trigger.*
- 7. Plan an alternate *positive response* to the same trigger before the next occurrence.
- 8. Continue until it is impossible to reach orgasm to the deviant fantasy.

It is prudent to test the process at the end of one month.

Some Caveats

The therapist must carefully supervise the above masturbatory reconditioning technique since it is totally dependent on self-report, the least valid form of information. During the first month, the excitement at success that comes with the technique is clearly visible in the client's attitude, behavior and demeanor, especially when he is unaware of being observed. Here again the need for *confirmation* from outside sources is essential.

A major danger with the technique occurs at the *first failure,* which is inevitable. Due to the perfectionism of the offender, this failure often becomes devastating and total, especially if an intervening month or more of success has occurred. Reassurance that this may happen and that, if it does, it is normal and important to the therapy process, helps the offender or private client through this perceived *disaster.*

Analysis of the reason for the failure will usually result in some new therapeutic knowledge and insight into the client and his personality, sensitivities and potential pitfalls. Here again, turning all *failures into positives* is a means of altering the negative perceptions and outlook of the client. All in all, the effort is worth the time and the problems associated with it. When done correctly, this form of masturbatory reconditioning rarely fails and will provide hope to the client that change really is possible.

15

A Holistic Approach to Treatment

As stated in the preface and in other sections of this work, one of the first things that we quickly learned about the treatment of the compulsive sex offender is that, in our experience, *conventional techniques usually fail.*

In 1976 the first sex offender treatment unit in New Jersey was opened (The Rahway Treatment Unit). In over a year or more of trying all the traditional therapy modalities, including psychoanalytic, behavioral, cognitive, Rogerian, nondirective and supportive techniques, therapists from all different backgrounds and professional trainings ended up deeply frustrated. Nothing at the time seemed to work. Even when we realized that confrontational techniques were necessary, they also failed to produce the positive overall effects that were necessary to treat the compulsive sex offender.

I quickly realized that psychotherapy alone would not work to produce a safe, healthy and, above all, happy individual. I finally found a positive and workable treatment attitude for sex offenders, which I term a *whole person* or *holistic approach.* Basically this means treatment not only for the *psyche* of the offender, but also for his body, mind and social being as well. Since, as can be seen from the list in Chapter 1, every facet of his being has in one way or another been negatively affected from an early age, so every facet of his life must somehow be involved in the treatment process. Over the years, the following elements of a holistic approach were formulated.

GROUP PSYCHOTHERAPY

The types of groups run were largely confrontive, but proceeded from different approaches, ranging from cognitive to behavioral. For a more complete discussion of this group psychotherapy process, see Chapter 9.

SEX EDUCATION

A *basic course* starts at approximately the sixth grade level. I found that sex offenders knew relatively little of the true facts about sexuality and could not pass a sex education test at this level. The basic course primarily covers:
- anatomy and physiology, both male and female;
- relational values and responsibilities;
- sexually-transmitted diseases, again emphasizing responsibility and positive prevention factors;
- body-image technique introduction;
- birth and its attendant facts and issues (birth control, male responsibility, decision-making regarding children, etc.

The *advanced course* continues from where each class in the basic course ended. At this point the course remains at grammar school vocabulary level and high school content level. The advanced course covers:
- body-image work (utilizing the Hartman-Fithian [1987] model;
- value formation and value change discussion and techniques (see Chapter 18 for specific content);
- film exposure and reaction homework;
- general rap sessions on any sexual topic that the class suggests;
- sharing of sexual developmental histories is also encouraged; and
- each individual chooses a book from a large sex education library to prepare an evaluative book report.

At this point, the offender is ready to enter the *sexual dysfunction level course*. The requirement for this level of the sex education program is that both prior levels (basic and advanced) were passed and that the individual's primary therapist recommends it. The sexual dysfunction course continues work in the area of distorted or deviant sexual values and how to change them. The focal topics include:

- sex guilt and how to deal with and overcome it;
- the skill of identifying one's own sexual dysfunction(s); and
- methods of preparing a treatment plan for dealing with and overcoming the identified problems.

The basic and advanced levels run the length of a normal U.S. college semester at the rate of three hours per week, while the advanced level course lasts at least a year and could go on for more than that, depending on the needs of the individual.

SOCIAL SKILLS TRAINING (SST)

As we previously concluded, one of the many failings in the sex offender is his low level of social skill and his inability to function socially with other individuals of his peer level. A terminal course that lasts about twelve weeks, the SST class is designed to help remedy this problem; it includes basic instruction in all aspects of social functioning. Role play that is videotaped and then played back immediately for group and therapist critique is crucial to the course. Areas covered include:

- how to meet someone and initiate a social conversation;
- how to successfully ask for a date;
- meaningful small-talk;
- how to say "No!" in an acceptable and appropriate manner;
- how to be *laughed at* and not take it personally (this includes being the center of attention in a group, making an error or acting silly and laughing at yourself with the group); and
- all other aspects of a normal adult social life that may be suggested by the class.

The "learning to be laughed at and not falling apart" segment of the class is extremely important due to the sensitivity and fear of failure or rejection that the sex offender brings into the class. Exercises are designed to promote laughter (sometimes to a hysterical level) and to prove to the individual that he will not die or collapse if this happens to him.

Changes are reported by feedback from the primary therapists. As their clients progress in this course the behavioral changes are visible in any situation where he interacts socially.

ANGER MANAGEMENT

This is another terminal course of approximately 12 weeks. The title of this course is misleading since participants are not taught to *control* their anger but rather learn how to *express* their anger appropriately.

As was previously discussed, where emotions are concerned, sex offenders are either impulsively explosive or suppress any emotional reaction whatsoever due to an immobilizing fear of punishment or rejection. Intellectual responses using emotional cues (love, anger, sorrow, hate, fear, sadness, sympathy, empathy, etc.) are meaningless in therapy since there is no ventilation of the original emotional reaction to an event, abuse, etc.

Sex offenders do not have to be taught emotions; they need to find a way to permit themselves to *feel emotion spontaneously* and to react emotionally towards individuals who precipitate the emotional response *as it occurs*. In this manner, projection and displacement of emotions on an innocent victim will hopefully be avoided.

This course permits and encourages emotional reactions to real events in the offender's life, either past or current:

- Each class member is asked to take the floor and to retell an emotionally-laden event, either in his past or in the present, and instead of repressing the emotions due to fear, allow them to spontaneously occur to whatever degree they are felt.

- Videotaping is utilized so that the offender can see himself emoting and so that the group and the therapist can offer feedback on the appropriateness of the emotional reaction and/or its degree.

As the offender becomes more comfortable with being an emotional human being and sees that his emotional response is appropriate and accepted by both peers and authority (the therapist), he is encouraged to begin taking risks in his daily life and to react emotionally when he chooses and/or when it is appropriate. Here again the primary therapists can see the effects of this course in their groups. Others in the offender's life also report the change from a nonreactive *"wimp"* to a more assertive and emotionally spontaneous person.

RELAPSE PREVENTION

Somewhere during the offender's treatment, the extremely important factor of relapse prevention must be dealt with. In institutional and correctional settings, a group setting for this course may be more appropriate and practical (due to numbers). However, in a community private practice it must still be dealt with but on an individual basis.

The main thrust of this course/discussion is to face reality about return to society or termination of treatment. The most important reality to present to the offender is that progress will not always remain upward and positive. In other words, *setbacks can and do occur.* Hopefully, these setbacks will remain at the thought or fantasy level and be reported immediately to the former therapist or a close friend or relative who knows the individual's past problems.

Offenders tend to think in extremes: everything is all or nothing, black or white, etc. Too often, without proper pre-release/termination preparation, the offender can encounter these feelings when first confronted with a setback:

- "Therapy didn't work."
- "I'm still the same old person."
- "What's the use, I may as well do it rather than go crazy thinking about it."
- "I can't tell anyone I'm failing and disappoint them when they put their faith and trust in me."
- "I can't let my therapist know I let him and my group down."

Being *forewarned* that this type of situation may occur, especially under pressure, stress, rejection or similar circumstances that triggered the original deviate reaction, is *essential.*

This course also aids the offender in preparing emergency and contingency plans for all sorts of unpredictable problems including:

- deciding whether to tell about his past in an employment interview;
- being fired when the employer finds out he is an ex-offender;
- rejection or distrust from a family member or loved one;
- discovering he can still be *turned-on* by his victim type (especially problematic in pedophiles and hebophiles);
- having problems with loneliness and not knowing where to meet new friends;
- needing support groups for a particular problem and not knowing where to find them (especially for A.A. [Alcoholics Anonymous] and N.A. [Narcotics Anonymous]);
- discovering his wife/fiancee/lover has been unfaithful while he was institutionalized;
- having his wife divorce him and take his children away upon his release;
- not being accepted as husband/father after a long institutionalization where the family learned to live without him.

This course, through consciousness raising about these problems and role playing situations that might occur, helps the individual to prepare for almost any eventuality.

VOCATIONAL RE-EDUCATION

For many sex offenders, it is impossible to return to their original profession/employment. This is especially true of teachers, priests, ministers, gym instructors, institutional personnel, police and correction officers, and other professionals exposed/convicted as sex offenders. This applies automatically to those involved with children or adolescents under their care.

For this very large group of offenders, a new life and vocation must be considered before release/termination and possibly new skills and requirements developed. Considering the *indecisiveness* of these individuals, it is dangerous to leave this task up to them alone. Vocational re- education provides a forum for group discussion and presentations of the possibilities that exist, especially in the specific area where the ex-offender intends living upon release from either an institution or correctional facility. Requirements, costs, training opportunities, vocational testing, etc., are all part of the knowledge that the course affords the pre-release offender. The final decision of a new vocation *remains solely his own.* If done in a group setting, the course may also afford previously unknown contacts and job opportunities.

SUBSTANCE ABUSE TREATMENT

For offenders with either a drug or alcohol abuse history, this type of group is a *must,* either in the community or in an institutional setting. Upon release from an institution, these affiliations must continue if successful re- entry into the community is the goal.

While alcohol and drugs *never cause the sexual deviation,* they quite often are contributing factors, usually affording the offender both the rationalization and the extra courage to perform the act.

Substance abuse groups help to dispel the *myth* that the abusing agent caused the sexual problem and to place full responsibility on the offender where it belongs. Since these are ongoing groups, senior group members can correct these distorted perceptions in new members. The fact that to be a member one had to be a substance abuser dispels the denial mechanism that therapists simply cannot crumble.

The *support* and *networking* elements of substance abuse groups like A.A. (Alcoholics Anonymous) and N.A. (Narcotics Anonymous) are their most important elements.

Feelings like *"I'm the only one this has ever happened to"* disappear almost immediately, and phone numbers are exchanged for those serious moments of temptation to dispel the "nobody cares!"cop-out (alibi, excuse, rationalization).

The difference in this group from the groups discussed above is that rather than being terminal it is a lifelong affiliation, although for many the frequency of attendance may decrease in time.

AFTERCARE

While the aftercare group has been mentioned before (see Chapter 10), it cannot be stressed enough. Abrupt release or termination from therapy, regardless of the amount of preparation, can be disastrous without providing some form of aftercare modality. In my opinion, this should preferably be a group format but can also be accomplished in individual therapy contact. Emergency telephone numbers to call on a 24-hour per day basis is also a necessary part of the aftercare modality.

In my experience, there is always some unfinished business and quite often a *secret* that was never divulged during formal therapy that is now causing problems for the released/terminated offender. In my years of conducting aftercare sessions for released sex offenders, I have asked the same question of each new member of the group:

- "Can you look me in the eye and honestly tell me that you never hid anything or kept any secret while you were in therapy?" I have *never*, in all of those years, had an affirmative response.

An open, accepting format for these types of "confessions," when they eventually occur (and they will!), must be provided if a new victimization and another failure are to be prevented.

16

Why Sex as the "Chosen" Deviation?

After a thorough analysis of the underlying dynamics of sexual offenses and the sexual offender, the question *"why sex?"* remains one of the most important treatment issues that may take many years to resolve.

For example, the *need to control* (either through force or seduction) can also be expressed in many non-sexual ways and behaviors. Money, position, power, fame, etc., are just a few of the means frequently used to control other people by individuals with a need to control who do *not* become sexual offenders. Certainly one's boss, a policeman in uniform, a judge in a courtroom, a Broadway or Hollywood star, a teacher, a father or mother in a family, an investor behind the scenes, and many, many other individuals in similar roles control people's lives daily *without* resorting to sex or sexually motivated behavior. Although control and all of the other sex offender traits can be clearly seen in other individuals who do not resort to sexual behaviors, the sex offender may find only *temporary* satisfaction in his deviant sexual behavior. Why this is his exclusive predetermined choice is still to be seen.

CHILDHOOD SEXUAL TRAUMA: CONSCIOUS /REPRESSED, ACTIVE/PASSIVE

In our discussion of the inadequate personality (in Chapter 2), the development of the repetitive compulsive sex offender was clearly seen and illustrated.

The essential and *differentiating factor* that separates the deny-ers, adjust-ers and accept-ers, who did not become compulsive sex offenders but who also overcompensated for their felt inadequacy, from compulsive sex offenders is the *sexual trauma*, conscious or repressed, that occurred to most, if not all, sex offenders and that was either never discovered, never reported or never properly treated. In Chapter 2, we have already seen a representation of the relationship between childhood personality, sexual crisis in adolescence, and normal or pathological sexual adjustment in adulthood (page 15, *supra*).

This trauma can occur at any age level but usually does not become traumatic until the child reaches *puberty,* when there is a major psychological change in the developing personality. This change consists of a *shift* from needing to please adults (parental figures) for acceptance, nurturance and love to needing to please and be accepted by *peers.*

Thus the adolescent *"Sturm und Drang"* (storm and stress) period for parents occurs during this time. The concern over what their peers think, feel and judge them by becomes a paramount issue for adolescents and determines their self-acceptance or rejection, their feelings of being normal or not normal, their ego strength and their self- esteem. Thus, whether they consider themselves to be normal and acceptable is not solely an internal judgment or decision, but is externally dependent on what others, especially peers, say. Locker room talk shapes their guilts and derogatory self-perceptions and the overall feelings of *inequality* that characterize the adolescent sex offender.

This psychological change also helps us to understand the *delay,* especially for boys, in reporting sexual abuse by adults that may have been going on for several years prior to adolescence. Were their involvement exposed (especially where boys are concerned), how could they remain in school with their peers? Permission from a higher authority is needed for the reporting to occur with some assurance that they will not pay a further price of peer rejection.

In Monmouth County, New Jersey, a program called *It Happens to Boys, Too!* has been able to overcome this barrier in a simple and direct manner. First, posters were put up on school bulletin boards (see illustration) with the above catch phrase and a hotline number. Concurrently, the posters were made into highway billboards. *Nothing else was done to promote the idea.* Calls from abused boys began coming in almost immediately and were then referred to proper agencies and therapists who had volunteered for the program. (The therapists, by the way, were *both screened and then trained*). When I interviewed one of the boys who responded and asked why it had taken him so long to report the abuse, his simple but profound answer was:

- *"I didn't know I was allowed to report a teacher. He told me I couldn't and then I saw the poster so I called."*

The pedophiles are well aware of this developmental characteristic (need for adult approval/acceptance) and take advantage of it on a regular basis. They find young pre- adolescent children whom they perceive as lonely, rejected and in need of acceptance and a relationship with a nurturing parental figure, usually missing from their lives.

The child victim, in turn, is so needy for this love and nurturing that he is willing to pay any *price* to keep it, once it has been experienced. No noticeable behavioral change may occur until adolescence and junior high school when the need for adult (parental) acceptance diminishes and is replaced by a need for acceptance from their peers.

The hebophiles are also aware of their chosen victim's needs (fear of peer rejection) and instill the concept of the sexual behavior remaining *"their secret."* Polaroid pictures and the threat that, if the hebophile is apprehended, these pictures will be seen by parents, friends, and teachers also cleverly uses this developmental knowledge.

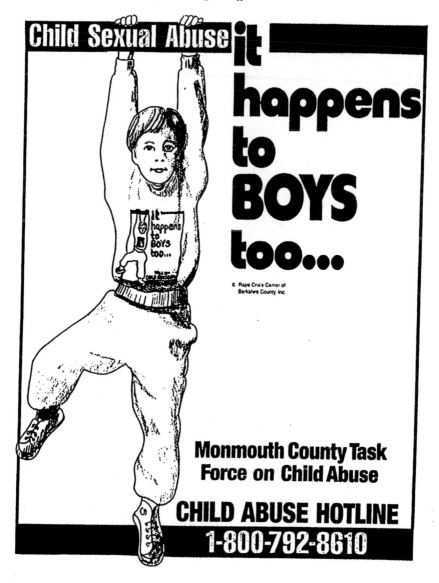

NEGATIVE EFFECTS OF UNREPORTED SEXUAL ABUSE

While it is obvious to state that unreported or unresolved sexual abuse will have negative effects, it is necessary to discuss the degree of this damage and the types of problems that *connect* to possible early sexual abuse.

The *trauma* occurs as the child enters adolescence and learns that sexual involvement with an adult, especially if homosexual, is neither accepted nor would it be tolerated by their judgmental and unforgiving peers. The adolescent may then either succumb to it (and become depressed, sometimes to suicidal proportions, turn to drugs and/or alcohol and, in general ruin their lives) or use every defense mechanism possible (denial, rationalization, even repression) to cope with their new dilemma. *Anger* at the adult offender, and also at their parents who should have protected them from the offender, now replaces *love,* and all blame is projected onto the adult (and all adults like the offender). A perception of victimization replaces the acceptance and love previously felt.

A *Catch-22* situation also exists for these victims: Should the relationship continue and become known, during this developmental period, the trauma will be even more severe and the guilt will be more deeply ingrained. Should the relationship end but remain undetected/unreported, the negative effects will remain and affect adjustment on all levels (self-worth, negative motivation, poor social interaction, isolation and either intellectual or physical overcompensation), especially the sexual level.

Sexual dysfunctions abound in these survivor groups, beginning at the onset of the trauma stage and continuing into adulthood. These sexual dysfunctions range from impotence to deviant arousal patterns, either pedophilic/hebophilic or sexually assaultive. The degree of the deviant fantasies or behaviors is usually directly proportional to the extent and depth of the original trauma and its duration.

If however, the child or adolescent gets into treatment with a qualified therapist, trained to deal with sexual abuse and its effects, and is able to put the experience into a proper and healthy perspective, the effects will be minimal and adjustment positive.

◆ NEGATIVE REACTIONS OF SURVIVORS OF SEXUAL ABUSE

A. DENY-ERS: Tend to repress the event. Their behavior abruptly changes but the true results of the trauma do not surface until later life, usually due to some triggering event (marriage, loss of employment, sexual failure, death of a loved one, etc.)

BOYS

◆ Often become satyrs to prove their manhood.

◆ If the behavior becomes pathological, they become sexually assaultive persons, especially if they were forcibly sodomized and interpreted this as being seen as a girl.

◆ End up referred for sexual-dysfunctions, especially impotence and premature ejaculation.

GIRLS

◆ Develop problems in their adult sex life, especially frigidity.

◆ See sex as dirty or disgusting; may become physically abusive parents without knowing why. Nudity is embarrassing and any arousal produces shame/guilt.

◆ End up referred for sexual dysfunctions, especially frigidity.

B. ADJUST-ERS: Usually have no negative effects since they:

◆ *Put all blame and responsibility on the abuser.*

◆ *Vent appropriate anger onto the abuser who molested them.*

◆ *Discuss what happened with their parents and friends.*

◆ *Ask for counseling or therapy if they feel the need.*

C. ACCEPT-ERS: Accept the abuse as deserved and their fault. As a result, self-image is damaged and the effects are long-lasting and sometimes permanent.

BOYS

◆ Repeat their abuse behavior on a same age child, almost ritualistically in order to reverse roles with the abuser.

◆ They now feel that they are the adult aggressor in control rather than being controlled.

◆ May show no other visible problems in their employment or social lives.

GIRLS

◆ Tend to prostitute, become promiscuous, or develop other self-punishing behaviors. Attempt to undo the abuse.

◆ Tend to marry aggressive, battering type (dominant) husbands.

◆ Tend to lose all goal motivation; isolate socially.

However, the adolescent *trust levels* will never return to pre-abuse levels.

It is logical to conclude that some form of *dysfunctional sexual behavior* results from sexual abuse, as other dysfunctions result from any other trauma. For example:

- A power trauma begets a power need and abnormal behavior in a related function of power. An example is the power-hungry politician or supervisor who goes beyond usual boundaries to obtain the so badly needed power.

- Physical abuse begets physically abusive behavior towards others, especially those who remind the abuser of himself at the time of his own abuse.

- Money trauma begets an obsession with wealth, and no matter how much the individual accumulates, it is never enough! Individuals born in poverty or during a period of war or depression, commonly show this symptomatic behavior.

In *incest*, there are more specific effects, as displayed in the relevant charts in this chapter.

WHEN TO SUSPECT SEXUAL ABUSE

As we discussed in Chapter 10, when the presenting problem of a new client includes *unwanted sexual thoughts or fantasies, deviant masturbation fantasies or overtly deviant behaviors*, it is logical and appropriate to consider sexual trauma in childhood or adolescence as a major causative factor.

It is quite rare during the intake session, for a client to identify childhood sexual trauma as the reason for his/her presenting problem. In addition, the trauma could possibly still be repressed.

What these clients do report is impotency, desire-phase deficiency, frigidity, compulsive and unwanted masturbation with disturbing fantasies, premature or retarded ejaculation problems and all other forms of sexual dysfunctions. When queried as to their thoughts about the cause of their problem, they simply have "no idea whatsoever; it just started."

At this juncture of the intake process, careful attention to the interviewing considerations in Chapter 9 will be helpful. The most important considerations are readiness and eliciting all of the

● **NEGATIVE EFFECTS OF INCESTUOUS ABUSE**

BOYS	GIRLS
◆ Repeat the offense in a ritualistic manner on younger siblings or sibling substitutes.	◆ Stress being adult. This change occurs as a sudden-onset occurrence.
◆ If forced, painful sodomy was involved, they often chose rape to deny their femininity and also to project their rage against their perceived nonprotecting mother.	◆ Overmakeup and overdress as seductive to satisfy their need for attention and sometimes for the father's continued approval.
◆ Display generalized rage at females throughout their lives that they cannot justify or explain.	◆ Start using their body and their looks for gain (learned from father).
◆ Tend to be aggressive and pain-producing in their sexual encounters.	◆ Become teases to boys and often to older men.
◆ Often have unresolved bisexual feelings and tendencies that frighten them and that they need to deny.	◆ Become outrageous flirts; partially to confirm their attractiveness, partially out of anger.
◆ Lose interest in school grades and often become school behavioral problems.	◆ Lose interest in school; want money, gifts, jobs, travel.
◆ Feel ambivalent towards the father; love and hate him at the same time.	◆ Consider the incestuous father their boyfriend or lover. This is usually the father's idea.
◆ As parents, fear having children since they might pass on their deviation or, even worse, become sexually abusive towards them.	◆ Become physically and emotionally abusive parents, but not sexually abusive. At times, this abuse ends in the death of a child.

nitty-gritty details of the trigger incident that began the dysfunction. An example will clarify:

☐ ROBIN *is a 22-year-old, attractive and intelligent graduate student who was recently married. The marriage lasted six hours, and she presently is separated and miserable. Robin was referred by her family physician with complaints of sexual anxiety resulting in frigidity, depression and fears that she was insane. Although quite anxious and emotional, she insisted on discussing the precipitating cause of her marital woes and related the following story.*

Robin met JESS in college and they were almost immediately attracted to each other. They dated for a full year and were then engaged. During the year and a half before their marriage they were affectionate and petted, but that was all that Robin would allow. Jess accepted her terms, based on her rigid Catholic upbringing, and patiently waited until they were married for sex. Following a large and extravagant wedding, they drove up to Niagara Falls for their honeymoon. They arrived around 11 p.m. and went straight to their suite.

Robin was the first to get ready for bed and went into the bathroom to change, closing and locking the door. She emerged in a new and proper nightgown, sat at the dresser and combed her hair. Jess went next and emerged from the bathroom nude and walked over to Robin. When she saw that he was nude she screamed "cover yourself up!" and went to the bed. She lay there staring at the ceiling and said "Do what you have to but don't expect me to enjoy it!" Jess was hurt, confused and angry all at the same time and yelled for her to get dressed since he was taking her home. They arrived back at their family homes around 4 a.m. without speaking a word during the entire trip. That was the last time Robin had seen Jess, more than three weeks ago.

There was little doubt that Robin had been sexually traumatized, although when asked directly about child sexual abuse, she denied it. In our second session, I felt she was more stable and less frightened or emotional and I opened by stating that she had done well in the first session and looked much better today. She smiled, and I then said, "Let's not worry about what happened at Niagara Falls right now. Instead, why don't you tell me about what happened to you as a child?" Robin immediately panicked and yelled, "I promised him I would never tell! He threatened to kill me if I did!" She then cried for some time, as the memories flooded in, and for the next several sessions she related her sexual abuse at the hands of her father from ages nine to 14. Her father was still alive and that made it more difficult for her to tell anyone what he had done. Therapy progressed quite rapidly after that and fewer than three months later, we were into couples' therapy with Jess. Therapy focused on desensitization to the male nude body, especially the male genitals. Sex therapy homework assignments were given when appropriate therapy progress had been made and, at the six month level, Robin and Jess consummated their marriage.

Months of time could have been wasted on what happened at Niagara Falls and we still would not have touched the real problem. Once the indicators of childhood sexual abuse are evident, that is where the therapy should focus, rather than on the presenting symptoms.

MASTURBATION AS AN ESSENTIAL RULER

Estimating progress levels in treating sex offenders, whether in an institutional setting or in private practice in the community, is a very difficult task. The credibility of their self-report is even lower than that of other client groups and the therapist must be careful not to be fooled. This is especially true where the therapist holds the keys to release from either an institution or from private therapy as a probation condition.

I have found careful analysis of the fantasies that the client uses for masturbation to be one of the best and most accurate rulers or measures of progress. Having the client *write out* these fantasies, as homework assignments, provides more details and exposes more deviant elements than if the client had to verbally describe the fantasy face to face with the therapist. It is also important not to read the client's homework in his/her presence, but to do so later and use the material gleaned for the next therapy session. Clients often try to *analyze* their therapist, and this is especially true of incarcerated sex offenders whose freedom relies on the therapist's evaluations. Once they realize that the homework will be read in their presence, a form of *censoring* occurs and the homework has less validity and meaning. The therapist specifically trained in this field will be able to find clues in the client's fantasies and writings that may never emerge in the formal therapy situation.

WRITING THERAPY

This form of adjunctive therapy is extremely useful with sex offenders in institutional or outpatient settings. Having them keep a journal (in bound notebooks rather than spiral, since they could easily remove pages from the latter) in which they record feelings, behaviors, interpersonal incidents and anything else that occurs between sessions, provides another valuable therapy resource. I even ask them to make an entry following each of our sessions, evaluating both of us and how they felt the session progressed. Sharing this journal with the therapist is strictly the offender's choice. Were it forced or conditional to the treatment process, it would lose much of it's value and could become a means for the client to manipulate the situation, which is always a major danger.

17

An Overview of Value Formation

Before any discussion of value change can be considered, we must first understand how values develop. Dealing with both offenders and victims of all ages made it necessary to formulate a descriptive, easily understood value formation progression. I have developed a five stage value development schematic that has worked successfully for me for the last 30 years:

FIVE STAGES OF VALUE FORMATION

Stage 1 — The Prisoner Stage (From Birth to 2 Years)

- All values are learned from parents and other adults in the child's home.
- Absolute obedience is necessary for acceptance and love.
- No comparisons are made at this stage.

Stage 2 — The Neighborhood Stage (From 2 to 5 Years)

- Friends, neighbors, relatives and others outside the home introduce new values.
- Comparisons by the developing child begin, and result in confusion and the first negative perceptions of parents and self.
- The first blame and guilt for failures also occurs during this stage.
- *Inadequacy* as a characteristic most likely begins in this stage.

Stage 3 — The Societal Stage (From 5 years to Puberty)

- School, religion and the law introduce additional values.

- Teachers, ministers, priests, scoutmasters, policemen, and other authority figures become new parent symbols and comparison intensifies.

- Value confusion is strong, especially when a behavior is acceptable at home and is not acceptable in school or vice versa.

- The need to please adults appears strongest in this stage and the child is therefore more vulnerable to seduction by the child molester, especially when the home is not fulfilling his or her needs.

- Parent-substitute interaction during this stage is critical to the mature and stable development of the child. Each needs to know what values the other is teaching and which values they are in disagreement with.

A child, like Bobby (see Chapters 4, 6, 7 and 9), who cannot speak his mind at home due to a tyrannical father, becomes confused in school when he is encouraged to be assertive and to speak his mind. Having opinions is acceptable and positive in school but forbidden and results in punishment at home. Which should he choose? On the one hand he still wants to *please* his father to earn acceptance and love, but on the other hand he wants to be his own person and the teacher and other authority figures in the community support and encourage this. Should he be disloyal to his father? The first time Bobby tried this new assertive behavior at home, it resulted in one of the worse beatings of his life. His feelings of being *different* are confirmed and magnified by this incident, since everywhere else he is expected to be someone that his father cannot accept. *Confusion* becomes the characteristic of this phase.

For others, like Mark (see Chapters 5, 7, 8 and 19), the confusion results from his school and community experience of observing other children receiving physical and emotional attention and comfort that was totally foreign to his home. His initial reaction is a feeling of being *undeserving*. However, when teachers and other authority figures offer him the same physical and emotional support outside of his home, he experiences the same confusion and feelings of being *different* that Bobby experienced.

The fact that this is the *pre-pubertal stage,* when physical and emotional changes begin, makes the reactions of the inadequate child even more exaggerated and affects the outcome of the next stage in a detrimental way.

With the completion of Stage 3, the child's need to please adults also ends. An *abrupt change* now occurs in the child's life.

Stage 4 — The Peer Stage (From the Onset of Puberty)

An abrupt psychological change occurs from the beginning of this stage until its completion, with the needs for acceptance and approval *shifting from adults to peers.* The initial result of this shift depends on the first three stages and how smoothly they were experienced.

Parents are most upset and disturbed about their children during this stage since they do not understand what is happening. Their formerly wonderful, obedient and loving child may now turn into a *monster* who is defiant, disobedient, argumentative and a constant source of irritation or even embarrassment.

In his/her quest for independence and personal identity, the child must now *break away* from the parents protection and direction and develop his/her own values, behaviors, decisions and even his/her own appearance (dress, hairstyles, etc.). The delusion that the awakening adolescent experiences is that these new decisions are his/her own, when in reality they are strongly influenced and dictated by peer standards and pressures. The fear of *being different* is magnified in this stage to it's greatest proportions.

Parents who, for status' sake, force their adolescent to attend high school in shirt, tie and jacket can expect problems of all sorts as a result, including defiance, torn or damaged clothing and hostility (bordering on rage). For the sex offender and his/her victims, *this stage is the most upsetting and leaves a lasting set of effects that must be dealt with in therapy.* The following problems may occur:

- Fears, self-doubts, confusion, shifts of loyalty, body-image problems and constant *testing* of both themselves and others.
- Communication abruptly stops and needs to be fostered regularly.
- Definitions of adult are fluid. Subtle help in deciding on a mature definition is needed but feared and/or rejected.

**• A SCHEMATIC REPRESENTATION OF THE MAGNIFIED EFFECTS
WHEN MOLESTATION OCCURS IN ADOLESCENCE**

BOYS

♦ If molested during stage 4 have a totally different reaction and experience. The need to be strong, macho and heterosexual dominates the male adolescent value system.

♦ A strong homophobic aura exists in male peer groups during this stage. In fact, it is my personal belief that this is the stage where true and intractable homophobia develops and remains with many males throughout their lives.

♦ Boys molested by older men during this stage cannot seek out support and comfort from their peers or from the majority of their male authority figure contacts, such as teachers, coaches, gym instructors, etc., or, most importantly, their fathers.

GIRLS

♦ If molested during stage 4 receive support, empathy and protection from both male and female peers as well as authority figures that they are involved with daily (e.g., their teachers).

♦ While the molestation is still traumatic, they do not feel rejected by their peers nor are they labeled or blamed for the occurrence, as frequently as boys are.

♦ They tend to report more readily and are much more motivated to become involved in therapy and then to get on with their lives. Naturally, there are exceptions to these reactions, especially when a girl is chronologically an adolescent but emotionally still a much younger child.

- Sexuality explodes and becomes a major focus. Indecisiveness and confusion about all aspects of sex dominate this stage.

- A war between old values (Stages 1, 2 and 3) and peer pressure occurs, and adds to the confusion.

- Guilt of all types flourishes and imprints.

- AIDS-phobia makes sexuality even more disturbing and confusing.

- Boy/girl expectations and demands separate more widely here than in any other stage.

Should sexual molestation occur during this stage, the effects will be *magnified* and become more *long lasting* than in any other stage. In addition, there is a major difference in peer reaction to an exposed molestation. These effects are displayed schematically in the accompanying diagram.

Two different types of examples of why boys *cannot* seek support from male authority figures follow:

☐ *While speaking to a high school senior class assembly on the effects of sexual molestation and the serious need for treatment when it occurs, I invited anyone who wanted to speak to me personally to remain after the assembly. (This had been pre-arranged with the school principal). Six girls and five boys remained, forming two small groups on opposite sides of the auditorium.*

In speaking to the girls first, I discovered that all but one were being incestuously molested at home. The sixth girl was molested by a male babysitter and never forgot the experience. All six were affected by the presentation and were now sobbing and allowing emotional reactions to pour out. There was little trouble in getting them all referred to therapists (this was pre-arranged with specialists in this area). The girls were willing to discuss their feelings with each other as a group and I networked them, since they all lived in the same general neighborhood.

The five boys were a totally different story. Although seen individually and confidentially, I learned that they were all involved with the same teacher. The time span of the molestations ranged from a minimum of one year to three years. None of the boys would consider reporting the problem or becoming involved in therapy. Their unanimous opinion was that if the story were ever revealed they would have to leave school, leave home and run away to a different state. They anticipated total rejection, putdown and labeling as "fags" or "queers" should their friends (peers) or other teachers find out.

The problem of the teacher was resolved with the school authorities without my revealing the facts or the identities of the boys. However, none of the boys (to the best of my knowledge) was ever treated for the molestations. Coincidentally, I was conducting a training seminar for all of the teachers, administrators and school board members of a different school district where a similar teacher-student sex scandal of several years duration had recently erupted. A male teacher had been arrested for his molestation of more than ten boys over a three year period. My function was to clarify and desensitize the situation. Still bothered and affected by the five boys in the first school, I decided to use a dramatic opening. I asked for a gym instructor or coach in the audience to stand up and help me with the presentation. A burly, muscle-bound football coach stood and said "Glad to be of service, Doc."

I knew I had the right person. I then instructed my "assistant" to be prepared to answer a question as quickly as possible without thinking or hesitation. He agreed. The question was: "What would you do if you discovered that one of the boys on your basketball team has been sexually involved with one of the other male teachers in the school?" I then snapped my fingers and the coach instantly replied "Kick the fuckin' fag off of the team and make sure that all of the rest of my boys knew about these two perverts!"

Needless to say, the five boys' predictions had been more than correct. A silence fell on the entire auditorium and I then thanked the coach for explaining why the molestations in his school had been going on unreported for several years.

Until we change these destructive values and reactions in adults, including parents and anyone entrusted with molding the minds and values of our children, sex offenders will have little trouble finding as many victims as their perverse desires require/demand. As mentioned in Chapter 16, Monmouth County, New Jersey's program *"It Happens to Boys Too . . ."* is a simple and effective method of attempting to correct this inequity between the way girl and boy victims (survivors) are treated by both peers and adults in authority that they deal with. Boys need to be told that it is *acceptable and proper* to report their molestations without being labeled, rejected and ostracized. Without programs of this type, the *merry-go-round of sexual abuse* will continue perpetually.

Stage 5 — The "I" Stage

All other stages and values are reexamined and decisions for adult life are made in this stage. Most adults either never reach this stage or continue throughout life to fluctuate between Stage 4 and Stage 5, depending on their emotional maturity, reaction(s) to trauma, need for approval and degree of ego strength.

Adolescents need to be made aware of this goal early in their development and must be encouraged to make decisions that will result in happiness. They must be urged not to settle for mere acceptance by peers, but aim for self-acceptance.

SEX = LOVE (LUV!)

Another insidious value, learned early in the life of both the sex offender, who was molested as a child/adolescent, and the child victim is that of *"sex = love."* How often has the challenge *"If you loved me, you'd ... "* been used by teenagers as well as adults to get a sex partner to do their will? Equally damaging is the molester's (both pedophile and hebophile) explanation of his/her sexual behavior as *showing love* to the victim.

As mentioned previously, in the United States more than in any other country, the damaging and destructive phrase *"making love"* has been used — due to embarrassment or puritanical needs — to justify or explain sexual behavior. Parents caught in the act of sex teach children from the earliest age that what they are doing is "making love," not having sex.

Love then becomes *sex* and vice versa, and physical disability, old age, etc., must mean that love no longer exists. Learned in the home, this becomes an easy tool for the molester to teach his victims all about adult lovemaking and to avoid the use of the dirty word "sex" at all costs. Even upon involvement in therapy, whether in a correctional setting or private practice, this *euphemism* acts as a defense mechanism against accepting the responsibility for the damage done to the victim. Hardened, repetitive compulsive rapists have stated in the beginning of therapy that they were only trying to show love to their victim (whether she wanted it from him or not!), or that they were hoping that if they satisfied her that she would then "love me."

VALUE CHANGE TECHNIQUES

No discussion of value change can be undertaken without first giving consideration to the important works of Professors Jane Loevinger and Lawrence Kohlberg. The reader is encouraged to take the time to research their all-important theories.

For the sex offenders and their victims that I have worked with, *changing a distorted, damaging or guilt-provoking value has been a seemingly impossible task.* As stated several times before, traditional or behavioral modification methods have not worked for me in this area and have produced levels of frustration that, for many clients, resulted in their quitting therapy. One of the most common guilt-provoking values found in these individuals is that of *masturbation guilt.* Regardless of the intellectual exercises that the patient goes through, when he next masturbates, the guilt returns and is perceived as even stronger. For years we struggled with this dilemma with no success until we developed the following explanation and homework assignment.

If one identifies the *unwanted behavior* and its underlying or associated *value(s),* but then jumps to the *change/confirm* column,

---

• VALUE CHANGE WORKSHEET USING MASTURBATORY GUILT AS A WORKING EXAMPLE

THE UNWANTED BEHAVIOR
→ Guilt following each masturbatory episode.

THE ASSOCIATED VALUE
→ Masturbation is dirty, sinful, abnormal, unhealthy.

THE SOURCE OF THAT VALUE AND ANY OTHER ASSOCIATED VALUES
→ I was caught masturbating by mother and punished; mother also stated that masturbation would lead to insanity and sterility. An associated mother-taught value was that "obedience = love."

THE CHOSEN NEW VALUE
→ Masturbation is normal and I don't have to give blind obedience to all of my mother's values to receive her love or to prove that I love her.

---

failure results most of the time and the above mentioned frustration ensues. Adding the *source of the value* column and carefully analyzing this area before attempting to change the value produces a positive result. When tested (for example by masturbating that evening) the guilt is gone, the frustration does not occur and the individual feels encouraged to attempt to change other, more difficult and entrenched values.

One phenomenon we have observed in this process is that in the *source of the value* column there are *embedded attached values* in addition to the obvious one that is being worked on. An example, at this point, will help.

☐ JOHN, *when 11 years old, was caught masturbating in the bathtub by his mother. With a stern and shocked look, mother admonished John, telling him that "he will run out of sperm and never have babies if he continues this dirty and disgusting practice." Although guilt-ridden and embarrassed for a short time, John continued with his masturbation but now experienced terrible guilt following each orgasm. Of course, he was careful to never again get caught by his mother. In working in therapy to change this value, John intellectually realized that he would not run out of sperm and that what he was doing was natural and not dirty. However, try as he might to change or eliminate the value, he suffered severe guilt after each masturbatory event. When John first used the above value change method, there was still no change in the guilt reaction. He was encouraged to search for an embedded attached value that might also have been learned from his mother (the source). When he came to the realization that his mother's love was dependent on his conforming to her values (total obedience) and that rejecting one of her values would result in his being rejected by her, he was able to see the total picture of conditioning that had occurred from his earliest memory. That evening his masturbation was the best and most pleasurable he had experienced and he fell asleep content with no guilt reaction.*

John was able to apply this same *source* method to rid himself of many other negative, limiting and guilt- producing values, and his progress in therapy accelerated.

It appears quite clear that beneath each surface value that cannot be changed through normal therapeutic methods there is an important person in the child's life who taught him that *"love = obedience."*

Bringing memories that contain this value to consciousness must be an essential part of the value change process and must be initiated early in the overall treatment process with both the offender and the survivor. These insidious values are imprinted at an early age and will remain there, affecting behavior and self-image to the point of sexual dysfunctions if not resolved. The damage is multiplied in cases where *pleasure results in guilt* and the persistent tug of war produces a level of mental anguish that easily leads to alcohol, drugs and other forms of escape from the pain.

There are many other distorted and destructive values that need to be identified when working with sex offenders or their victims.

"Sex = love" and *"obedience = love"* are two defective values that most frequently affect the adult behavior of this group. The remaining list of destructive values includes:

- Love = slavery,
- Acceptance = conformity,
- Sex = pain,
- Pleasure = evil,
- Love = punishment,
- Free will = delusion,
- Deviancy = genetic,

- Silence = loyalty,
- Love = loyalty.

The list is endless. However, the value change technique is the same for any distorted, justifying or deviant value that is identified.

18

Self-Confrontation and Resistance in the Compulsive Sex Offender

In most compulsive sex offenders, regardless of the therapeutic setting, *resistance* is most often the primary barrier to therapeutic insight or change.

This has certainly been true in my experience with hospital, correctional, and private settings. The need to develop a method of eliminating this barrier is paramount to any successful treatment. Part of the reason for this resistance is the compulsive sex offender's major use of *denial* as a primary defense mechanism. The more intense the guilt he/she is experiencing, the stronger the *denial* and consequently the greater the resistance.

Since therapist confrontation methods did not work with these most resistant cases, we had to develop a *pre- therapist confrontation method* that the clients could do by themselves. The result was called "Now Therapy: A Method Of Self-Confrontation for More Frightened and Resistant Cases."

After many, many frustrating hours of trying to break down the resistance and minimize the denial, the task appeared hopeless, until one patient made the following casual remark in the heat of an emotional outburst "How can I admit something to you I haven't even admitted to myself!" Following this session, I did a quick survey of other highly resistant clients and found they all had the same problem.

THE FIRST "NOW" THERAPY SESSION

While pondering how to tackle this perplexing dilemma, a fortuitous incident occurred. In the sex education courses I conducted, an important module in the advanced section was the Body-Image exercises of Hartman and Fithian (1987). For many reasons, I had to modify the original technique to the following format:

- The exercise is conducted in a group setting, utilizing a tailor's three-paneled mirror.
- The client stands before the mirror in the nude and touches each part of his body, from the top of his head to the soles of his feet.
- As he touches each part, he describes how the part *feels* to him, whether he *likes* the part or not and why.

When this exercise is completed, the client is told to do the following three tasks:

1. Rate the body you are looking at on a 0-100% basis, comparing it to your peer group and considering your age. Once he makes a determination he is told "now explain the reasons for your rating."

2. Choose just one part of the body you are looking at that you would like to change. Once the part is chosen he is asked to "explain the reason for your choice."

3. Choose just one part of the body you are looking at that you would like to take with you to a totally new body. Once the part is chosen he is asked to "explain the reason for your choice."

The answers to these three follow-up questions alone are significantly diagnostic. The therapist must pay close attention, especially to the *reasons* for the choices.

When this part of the exercise is completed, the client turns around and faces the group. Each group member is then asked by the therapist to answer the same three questions about the body they are looking at and to give his own reasons for his choices. When this is completed, the client is asked if his rating percentage is still the same or if it has now changed. In more than 75% of the cases, the group's evaluation and rating alters the body-image perception of the client. Most frequently, the rating increases, but there are cases (especially in narcissistic personality types) when the re-evaluation results in a lower rating.

☐ *The day after* MARK *took his turn doing the body-image exercise, he asked to see me in my office. He appeared quite anxious and stated, "That sex ed thing last night really affected me. I didn't want to leave the mirror. It just wasn't enough. I would have liked to talk to the guy in the mirror about himself, his behavior and other things, not just about his body." Since the therapy room was available at that hour, I asked Mark if he would like to go and continue the session. He readily and happily agreed. Back in front of the mirror he began, "Well, I guess you are a nice guy . . . and people tend to like you and want to be your friend" — then a silence of over 20 minutes, followed by: "But you're not worth shit!"*

I then asked him to tell the man in the mirror why he felt that way about him today, without using anything from his past. Another lengthy silence followed, after which he stated, "I can't." I then asked him to reappraise the man in the mirror and he said, "Well, maybe you're not so bad after all." Smiling, he left the mirror and said that he felt as if a thousand-pound weight had been lifted from his shoulders.

Excitedly, he told his group what had occurred during their next session; they all wanted to try the technique. Instead, a small committee was formed to develop the format and procedures for such a group. Concurrently, I presented the technique to the treatment staff of the institution for their appraisal and asked them to refer clients who fit the same resistant-to-change category.

The final technique that emerged thus pivoted on *self- confrontation* in a private and safe setting where no one could hear or observe. Since *"admitting it to myself"* appeared to be the key, it also became the primary technique.

Expecting the client, no matter how motivated, to bare all in the first session was senseless and so a slow, gradual approach to complete openness had to be built into the system. Since *identity* was also an issue, this became the approach to the problem. The client's first assignment was to stand in front of a full length mirror (in his bedroom or alone in a therapy room prepared for the technique) and to *distance* himself from the person in the mirror by using the second person "you" rather than "I" in all of his statements.

After several months of experimenting, two other elements were incorporated: *the technique worked best when (1) the client was in the nude* and *(2) the client spoke aloud.* Upon first presentation of the technique to a small group of professionals with whom I was associated at the time, there was some immediate concern and criticism about using nudity with sex offenders. In order to deal with these concerns, several other methods were tried. Shorts, underwear, bathing suits, etc., were all tried and the technique failed. Defenses remained stronger than ever and blocking occurred. The offenders themselves felt the discomfort and returned to the original method.

Where the second condition is concerned, thinking or mental confrontation (as opposed to speaking aloud) also failed. Apparently all of the lies, fantasy materials and distortions that the sex offender uses daily kept intruding. But, if the client looked himself in the eye and spoke out loud, *it became impossible to lie.* He would actually interrupt himself and confront any attempted lie or distortion, such as minimizing.

An unexpected bonus also occurred in all clients using the technique: there was a noticeable increase in self-confidence, although no direct work had been done in this area. Others in the sex offender's life (parents, wives, children, work supervisors, etc.) reported the change, as did the client himself.

What appears to happen is as follows. For most of his life, the compulsive sex offender has been out of control or at least *perceived* that others controlled all of his life and decisions, whether parents, teachers, friends, employers, wives, lovers, even his children. In this technique it is *impossible* not to accept credit (that could never be tolerated before) for any change, insight, or faced experience. Once motivated to attempt the technique, the technique and the individual take over, and most of what occurs is unplanned, regardless of the amount of rehearsing that precedes the actual session.

The greatest fear, in a majority of cases, is facing the fact that he is a sex offender. Standing there telling his *"friend"* in the mirror that he is a sex offender has a permanent shock value that does not disappear.

THE COMMUNITY OR PRIVATE PRACTICE "NOW" TECHNIQUE

Converting the "Now" technique for use in private practice in the community was a simple task. The client is instructed to perform the technique at home in the privacy of his bathroom or bedroom in front of a full length mirror. It is essential that *no one else be present during the exercise.* This is a means of eliminating any possible defensive reaction based on what others would think, feel, etc. It is also strongly suggested that an inexpensive cassette tape recorder be placed on the floor by the mirror to record the session, since it has been our experience that clients will defensively *forget* parts of the session that were highly sensitive or traumatizing. The client is told to listen to the tape within 24 hours and to note, for himself, what he hears on the tape that he had forgotten (re-repressed). While the tape is strictly for the client's use, it has been my experience that many clients will bring a tape or two to the following session to share with the therapist.

When used in an institutional situation, the "NOW" technique should either be continued after release and discussed in follow-up contacts, such as an aftercare program, or be initiated when the need arises if the released individual had never used the technique before.

CAVEATS

Several caveats must be discussed.

- The session should always be at least audiotaped, where videotaping (the ideal method) is not available. The most traumatic and shocking revelations and/or accusations can be re-repressed following a session; thus the need for a permanent and objective record. Instructions should carefully explain that this taping is for the client, not for the therapist, in order to prevent *performance-oriented* sessions.

- The therapist must ensure that these sessions do not become *self-punishment* sessions, a real danger with the compulsive, guilt-ridden offender. His negative self-image is bad enough when he starts therapy and care must be taken that this negative image does not become intensified. Weekly reports from the client on the self-confrontation sessions are used for this purpose and the client himself will often volunteer a tape of a session that he was either pleased with or that disturbed him. Listening to the tapes in his presence become highly therapeutic (and revealing as well) since they all run a *commentary* on their performance as the tape plays. This playback session also affords the therapist an opportunity to provide guidance for future sessions through the use of subtle suggestion or highly directive suggestion, depending on the circumstances.

- *Mirrors* then become a major homework assignment with the content left entirely up to the individual. The reason for this is that the current issues in his therapy may be overshadowed by an immediate and pressing problem in his life. Should he feel the obligation to do what the therapist told him, he may use his directed homework as a means of avoiding his daily life problems.

- As the client becomes more comfortable with self- confrontation, the therapist, either in an individual or group setting, can begin to become more directly confrontive with him.

The overall major benefit is a new self-confidence and a lessening of the almost complete dependence these clients have on the therapist. More risks will be taken and more new behaviors attempted. Here, as in all therapy modalities, *nothing succeeds like success.*

The following example concerns a man who had been in therapy first with a well-known therapist in the community and then in an institutional setting. After his release the following occurred:

☐ JUAN *was a 35-year-old rapist who was well-liked at the treatment center. From his entry into treatment he appeared open, cooperative and willing to tell all. Progress in therapy was rapid and the insights developed in his case appeared to logically and firmly explain his behavior. Juan had begun his sexual problem history with flashing (exposing himself) to younger girls in his neighborhood and school. This behavior began at age 11 and continued through early adulthood, when he was first arrested. Juan was sentenced to one year of probation with the condition of weekly psychotherapy, and quickly was promoted to bi-weekly, monthly and finally terminated (all in six months). The flashing continued both during his treatment and afterwards, but he was not arrested again until his first rape of a young adult female.*

Juan was married with three children at the time and had a steady job where he was used and abused. Rarely did he express a negative emotion, and he appeared frightened of anger. The reasons he allowed himself to be used and taken advantage of were never discussed in his probation therapy sessions. Once institutionalized, his progress was rapid and convincing. In a relatively short period of four years, he earned his parole and was enrolled in the aftercare program that I conducted. From the start, I had a gut reaction that something was wrong but could not identify the problem. He smiled at anything and everything and appeared to be adjusting well to his return to society. He reported some minor problems with reestablishing his role as father and head of the household but since his children were adolescents, this did not appear to be unusual. One year after his release, almost to the day, Juan was arrested for flashing two young girls at a crowded shopping center in midday. He was immediately apprehended and released on his own recognizance with a court date in one month. He arrived at his next aftercare session depressed and needing to take the floor. After telling the group what happened, he insisted that he had no idea why it occurred and it made as little sense to him as it did to anyone else.

After having him begin the "Now" self-confrontation exercises, the following individual session took place.

Juan reported that standing in front of the mirror and talking to himself produced an unexpected anger outburst. He told the man in the mirror that he was "no good, rotten and deserved to go back to jail!" I immediately sensed that he was hiding something and kept asking for more until he finally told me that while confronting himself in the mirror, he suddenly remembered being sexually abused when he was a small child.

Juan's father deserted the family when he was only seven years old and his mother, who spoke very little English, could not find work. The rent was due and they were evicted. His mother's only recourse was to ask friends to take them in. After two or three of these short-term visits, she found a woman who said she would let them live there as long as they liked as long as Juan's mother would do some housework, cook and look after her two teenage boys so she could go to work. Juan's mother happily agreed and they moved in. Juan had to sleep with the two boys while his mother shared the only other bedroom with their benefactor. During the second night, the boys undressed themselves and then Juan and introduced him to his first sexual experience. Their penises looked gigantic to him and the boys made fun of the "little-finger" he had between his legs. They then made him masturbate each of them and threatened to kill him and his mother if he told anyone. After a week of abuse, Juan went to his mother and told her the whole story in Spanish. She answered "Juan, we have nowhere to go! Please, be a good boy and do what the two brothers ask you to do or we'll be out on the street." Disappointed, confused and angry, Juan submitted to the abuse which eventually escalated to painful sodomy. After the first sodomy experience, Juan considered himself a "Puta" (female prostitute) and his self-image totally changed. He reasoned that since he was sexually attractive to the two boys, he must have appeared or acted feminine and that was why they "used him as a girl."

In all of his therapy, both individual in the community and group in prison, he never related this story and its connection to his flashing (his need to be accepted as a male, even with his small penis) or the anger at his mother that led to the rape behavior. Juan continued doing the "Now" technique at home and even taught it to his wife and to his children. Today they are a happy family, travel together and have long, meaningful discussions. Juan could never relate to his wife or children in this way prior to the self- confrontation. At work, he no longer is the whipping boy and asserts his rights with everyone including his employer. The result has been a raise in pay and better working hours.

"Now" or self-confrontation must become a way of life and a daily exercise for Juan and others. In the morning, it should be used to set realistic goals for the day, and in the evening, to evaluate the day on both a positive and critical level. The *balance* is the important factor, as is the fact that the client now becomes his own therapist and takes charge of his life.

In formal therapy, the results of these self-confrontations are discussed to be sure that they are balanced and that the defective goal-setting pattern has not returned.

19

Conclusions

In all of our training sessions, a pretest is used to raise the consciousness levels of the participants (see Chapter 1). A primary question and concern during this test revolves around the qualifications of the individual wanting to treat or already treating sex offenders. Besides a degree or certification, there are personality requirements that are of utmost importance; thus the question: *"Of all the many required traits and characteristics of the intended sex offender therapist, which is the most important and most frequently absent?"*

Rarely is the correct answer obtained in the pre-training questionnaire. The most important trait or characteristic of the intended therapist for this group, in my opinion has always been: *comfort with sexuality; his/her own and that of others.* An example will clarify the importance.

☐ BRIAN, *a 12-year-old survivor, is being interviewed by a middle-aged female psychologist for the first time after his sexual molestation. They are in her office, with Brian sitting next to her desk and she facing him. Her first question to Brian was: Brian, tell me what happened." Brian then asked if it was all right to tell her what the teacher did to him, since she was a woman. She replied, "Of course it is. You can tell me anything you want. Use your own words." Brian then replied, "He (Brian's 5th grade teacher) took me into the cloak room and made me suck his dick!"*

Immediately, the therapist swiveled in her seat to face the desk, lowered her head and began furiously writing. Brian glared at her with obvious anger and said, as he got up and left the office, "You lied to me!" When questioned later about the incident, Brian stated that he did not want any of that therapy stuff. He never returned to therapy.

Since this was a supervised session and was videotaped, the supervisee was asked what she felt had happened and she replied that she was "shocked at the boy's filthy language!"

Unfortunately, this was Brian's first contact or experience with therapy and *also his last.* He refused to return to the clinic or to see anyone else about his molestation and became a consistent behavior problem in school, ending up involved with the juvenile authorities.

Not only may *language* shock the naive or untrained therapist, but also the *content* of the sexual behaviors themselves. Remember the incident of the young boy who masturbated the elephant? (See Harry, chapter 5.) Definitely not your everyday sexual behavior.

Beside specialized training (which is a *must*), it is my opinion that attendance at an S.A.R. (sex attitude restructuring) seminar or course is a necessary prerequisite to becoming a therapist for either sex offenders or survivors. Supervision with an experienced and qualified sex therapist becomes the next necessary experience. For some trainees, therapy with a certified and trained sex therapist may also be necessary to deal with their own personal issues, especially those that could affect their treatment of clients adversely.

NEED TO SEPARATE PERSONAL MORAL CODE

The ability to separate your own personal moral and religious values from the therapeutic experience is an absolute necessity in working not only with offenders but also with survivors.

If the sex offender can *shock* the therapist with graphic descriptions of his sexually perverse behaviors, he will use this as a *control mechanism* (his primary need) to change subjects or to end sessions that are becoming uncomfortable or anxiety provoking. Similarly, the survivor constantly *tests* the therapist before revealing his most horrible experience (subjectively perceived). If, as in Brian's case, the therapist reacts with shock, revulsion or disgust, that can become the survivor's justification to quit therapy and never have to face his most dreaded memories.

In cases of *homosexual molestation* of long duration, the male survivor is often confused as to his present sexual identity. A major concern in exposing himself to the therapist may be revealing that he enjoyed many of the sexual encounters and still is fantasizing and/or masturbating to memories of these past experiences. Additionally, he may be feeling attracted to other boys his own age or to men who remind him of his abuser. The therapist must take great care not to reveal his/her own feelings on this subject, especially if he/she is opposed to a homosexual lifestyle.

Training, in this instance, will aid the therapist in helping the survivor to make *his own decision* as to a sexual preference or lifestyle, including the possibility of a *bisexual option* rather than either extreme.

Females molested over long periods of time may choose not to marry but rather to live with someone. Here, again, the therapist's own moral preferences and/or convictions should not enter the therapeutic situation.

NO JOB IS WORTH HARMING YOURSELF OR YOUR FAMILY

This is an appropriate juncture at which to consider whether an individual choosing to work in this field (which I refer to as the "cesspool of sex offenses") can afford the *price.* Let us consider several areas:

- Listening to the sordid and often horrifying details of the sex offender's own life and his deviant behavior can be too much for some individuals.

- Having to remain *neutral* on subjects of moral values and decisions can affect the personal life of the therapist.

- The *depressive* quality of daily encounters with human suffering at levels never before experienced or even imagined can affect the emotional life of the therapist.

- Coming home daily from the emotionally charged atmosphere of working with offenders can alter the therapist's reactions to his partner and family.

- Some individuals are unable to distance themselves from their work sufficiently to prevent problems being brought home and *dumped* on family members, including wives and children.
- There is a constant danger of becoming *overly protective* and restrictive with one's children after working daily with the child molester group.
- The effects of *keeping secret other sex crimes*, including sex murders, which are covered by confidentiality, can and does effect the therapist without a prepared support system of his/her own.

The bottom line is that not all therapists are emotionally equipped to work in this field and that is not a reflection on their professional ability or competence.

REDEFINING PROFESSIONALISM: TOO-CLOSE-TO-HOME CASES, PERSONALITY CONFLICTS, AND KNOWING WHEN TO ASK FOR HELP

Individuals choosing to work in this or related fields must first redefine traditional concepts of professionalism. The old precepts of the three piece suit therapist with multiple degrees, diplomas and certificates hanging on the wall does not, by itself, qualify anyone for this field, nor does it bode success.

Anyone wanting to be successful in this endeavor of treating the compulsive sex offender must throw away traditional concepts and techniques, and become a *pragmatist.* What succeeds in this field is whatever works, and that changes from one offender to another. Even with the basic similarities in personality traits that we listed in Chapter 1, the *individual differences* of the sex offender dominate the overall picture.

Flexibility is a major requirement for any treatment program that is to succeed. The techniques and principles I used and followed in 1967 with the first treatment program no longer worked in 1976. Similarly, techniques devised in 1976 no longer work in 1990, and so on.

THE PROGRAM MUST CHANGE WITH EACH NEW GROUP OF OFFENDERS ENCOUNTERED AND MUST FIT THEIR INDIVIDUAL NEEDS

When facing each new group of offenders, the therapist must make adjustments, such as dropping all professional jargon and college level vocabulary, which puts distance between the offender and the therapist. In addition to these exterior changes the therapist must also alter his/her way of thinking. Constant *self-monitoring* and *peer supervision* must be an integral part of the program. Cases that come *too close to home* or that pose a serious *personality conflict* from the first meeting must be transferred to another therapist to avoid disastrous results for everyone.

If, for example, the school, neighborhood and age of the victim that the offender molested is identical or nearly identical to the therapist's own child, it is unrealistic to expect *objectivity* from that therapist.

Similarly, if the therapist experienced a sexual assault in his own family or that of a close relative, cases that are similar to that assault should not become part of his/her caseload. Certainly, a therapist should not treat the rapist who raped his wife (although I know of a case where that was attempted, with disastrous results for both the client and the therapist) or who molested one of his/her children.

Where personality conflicts are concerned, there will always be cases that from the first meeting (especially if the details in the individual's record have been read beforehand) result in immediate dislike and anger/rage toward the client. The therapist must be professional enough in such cases to decline the assignment. Two specific examples from my own experience will clarify:

☐ *When young and new to the field, I was assigned to do an evaluation that would result in a recommendation to the court on a particularly violent and sadistic sex offender. I made the error of reading the police investigation from cover to cover, prior to seeing the offender. The report included color photographs of the autopsies of three young children that the offender had sexually raped and then mutilated, cutting their bodies into multiple parts and disfiguring the faces. The pictures and autopsy description made me ill.*

Fewer than fifteen minutes after finishing the report, the offender was escorted into my office and my immediate urge was to attack and harm the man. I excused myself and went to my supervisor and told him I was unable to do a fair and objective evaluation. He threatened me with suspension for "acting unprofessionally" and insisted that "a good professional can handle anything and anyone." Young and arrogant, I stood my ground and went over his head to his supervisor, who agreed with my position and assigned the case to my supervisor.

I learned two things from that case:

- A good professional knows when he or she is in over their head and when to say "no."

- One should never read an investigative report on a case *until* an evaluation is completed and impressions recorded. I still advise new individuals to the field to do this.

KNOWING WHEN TO ASK FOR HELP

A second opinion is also of vital importance in working with sex offenders. *Gut reactions* can be important clues that something is not right with a case. When any doubt arises, consultation with another individual in the field is the professional course of action.

False professionalism may dictate total independence and autonomy in all cases. The results can be disastrous for the offender, the therapist or for potential new victims. Where possible, the consultation or second opinion should be with a therapist of the opposite sex. Why? For many reasons, *sex offenders behave and react differently with men and women depending on their proclivities and needs.*

Rapists, for example, tend to be less aggressive or challenging with men than with women. It is much easier for a female therapist to trigger their anger and rage. I would never make a final decision as to readiness for release of a S.A.P. (sexually assaultive person) from treatment without first exposing him to several months of contact with a female therapist, trained to *trigger* male anger and rage reactions.

Sex offenders tend to identify with male therapists who satisfy their needs for paternal acceptance, affection and love. If such an offender is with a supportive, gentle and highly positive therapist for a long time, he should concurrently be working with a confronting, strong and more challenging female therapist. This is true for both rapists and child molesters.

Child molesters who have been working exclusively with a warm, supportive female therapist (substitute mother figure) should be exposed to a male therapist as well to provide a role model and because the child molester generally fears men more than women. Being accepted as his old passive and frightened self will not ensure success in the child molester's treatment.

In general, where feasible, co-therapy works much better with sex offenders than being in long term treatment with one person.

TRANSFERENCE AND COUNTER TRANSFERENCE

In no other form of treatment are the concepts of transference and counter transference as important and as frequent an occurrence. Due to the sex offender's desperate need for acceptance and love, *transference* occurs almost in every case.

A simple definition will suffice for our purpose here:

Transference is the phenomenon of projection of feelings, thoughts and wishes, *on the part of the client,* onto the therapist, who has come to represent an object (person) from the patient's past. (Wolman, 1989, p. 352)

Transference can be both positive and negative, can refer to identification, libido, love, sibling, group or affect. The main concern for the therapist or anyone else working with the offender is to be able to *recognize* the transference when it occurs and not to interpret it as the offender's real feelings for the therapist.

Counter transference is the phenomenon of projection of feelings, thoughts and wishes, *on the part of the therapist,* onto the patient who has come to represent an object (person) from the therapist's past. (Wolman, 1989, p.78)

The danger here is obvious. If the therapist is not aware of the counter transference occurring, he/she can become omnipotent, retaliatory, controlling and *use* the patient to satisfy his/her own unresolved needs.

Both of these phenomena are complicated and should be studied separately from this work. They are mentioned here only to indicate the need for constant *peer review and supervision.*

ANY FAILURE IS HIS, NOT YOURS

Too often, therapists working with sex offenders accept responsibility for the failures of the offender, especially if he is released from treatment and recommits his deviant behavior. This reaction on the part of untrained therapists reflects the old and constant misperception that *therapists treat patients.*

The longer one is in the field, the more obvious it becomes that *patients treat themselves* and that the therapist, counselor, parent or friend, is only a coach or guide during the therapy. A football or basketball coach does not go out onto the field and win or lose the game; the players do, and the same applies to therapy. The most important concept to learn from the beginning is that *all change comes from an inside motivation and need, not from outside pressure, pleading or cajoling.*

No change will occur until the client wants it to. This is more true for the sex offender than for any other group I have worked with. As long as the offender feels unworthy or undeserving, nothing will occur that is perceived as positive. If a positive occurs, he will destroy it. Too often, that is exactly why a failure occurs: *the offender does not feel that he deserves to be happy or successful and deliberately (although on an unconscious level) sets himself up to fail.*

Years ago in the original treatment unit at the then Rahway State Prison, I used the phrase *"can't stand prosperity,"* as the major diagnosis in most returnees or failures. Usually, everything was going *too well* for the offender, and past, unresolved guilts tortured him to the point of such discomfort, he had to find a way to return to prison "where he belonged" and felt comfortable.

Regardless of how well trained and intentioned the therapist may be, the content of what the client exposes is always in his control. No matter how sure we may feel that everything has been exposed and resolved, it is too often the case that a secret remains that is simply too terrible to tell anyone. Placing all responsibility on the offender, where it belongs, is a major therapeutic element, and applies to returning to deviate fantasies and behaviors as well. The offender's failure is his and not the therapists.

FINAL THOUGHTS

Thirty years of "swimming in the cesspool of sex offenses" has taught me conclusively that *sex offenders can be successfully treated.* All the same, it would have been much easier had specialized training been available in 1967, or even earlier in 1961, when I began working with children and adolescents who had either committed sex offenses or were the victims of them.

The major purpose of this work has been to help prevent other individuals new to this field from making the same mistakes that I and other therapists working with me have. My experience has convinced me beyond doubt that there are techniques that work with offenders, and others that definitely do not.

The book has not pretended to be all-inclusive. Supervision is still paramount, regardless of the amount of knowledge that one accumulates. What one knows is much less important than what one does not know. Therefore *questions* play a major role in all training and learning. Trainees sitting passively in training sessions, afraid to ask questions due to image problems, remains the most difficult barrier for a trainer to overcome. I encourage my trainees to write their questions in disguised handwriting and leave them unsigned where the trainer can find them and include them in the training. This is especially true when line personnel are placed in the same training session with their supervisors. However, those who really want to learn will overcome this problem.

Besides the constant push for specialized training that I have included in the book, the *caveats* come next in importance. While treating sex offenders is necessary and urgent, it is not worth trying to help one offender at the cost of damaging another individual (the therapist, counselor, etc.). While the successful conclusion to a treatment case can be both rewarding and professionally satisfying, the cases that we don't reach and who carry on unhappily in their deviant lives can be depressing and discouraging. There must be a balance in the life of the helper for it to make sense. A strong family life, support at home and from professional colleagues, friends to talk to and ventilate with, tons of love to replace the pain; all of these are essential to maintaining a healthy helper.

If I have been able to help just one offender from recommitting, I have succeeded in my goal and it has been worth all the grief and pain. Just consider the numbers: if I help one rapist from recommitting, then at least 12 to 25 potential victims have been spared.

If I help just one child molester then as many as 100 child victimizations may have been prevented, as well as *their* future victims if their molestation is not successfully resolved.

SUCCESSFULLY TREATING SEX OFFENDERS IS A MAJOR SEXUAL ABUSE PREVENTION TASK AND MORE NECESSARY THAN EVER WITH TODAY'S RISING VICTIM RATES.

Appendix

☐ *1. All sex offenders, regardless of offense, have major personality traits in common.* **TRUE**

☐ *2. All sex offenders were themselves sexually victimized as children and this explains their behavior.* **FALSE**

☐ *3. Sex offender pathology can be genetically linked.* **FALSE**

☐ *4. Pedophiles and hebophiles have the same characteristics and prognoses for treatment success.* **FALSE**

☐ *5. Fixated pedophiles may appear normal in their social, work, and interpersonal functions.* **TRUE**

☐ *6. Hebophiles and incestuous fathers have many traits in common and a similar (and more positive) prognosis for treatment success.* **TRUE**

☐ *7. The King-of-the-Castle syndrome is a major distinguishing characteristic of incestuous fathers.* **TRUE**

☐ *8. Supportive and non-confrontational treatment techniques work better with sex offenders than other treatment modalities.* **FALSE**

☐ *9. Psychotherapy itself will produce positive results with sex offenders.* **FALSE**

☐ *10. Following their victimization, victims of sexual abuse have many traits in common with sex offenders.* **TRUE**

REFERENCES

Burgess, Anthony. 1963. *A Clockwork Orange.* New York: Norton.

Groth, A. Nicholas. 1979. *Men Who Rape: The Psychology of the Offender.* New York: Plenum.

Hartman, William E., & Fithian, Marilyn A. 1987. *Body/Self Image.* Los Angeles, California. Sensate Media Service.

Krafft-Ebing, Richard von. 1922. *Psychopathia Sexualis.* Brooklyn: Physicians & Surgeons Press.

Loevinger, Jane. 1976. *Ego Development.* San Francisco: Jossey-Bass.

Kohlberg, Lawrence. 1969. Stage and sequence: The cognitive development approach to socialization. In D. Goslin (Editor), *Handbook of Socialization Theory and Research.* Chicago: Rand McNally.

Masters, William H., Johnson, Virgina E., & Kolodny, Robert C. *Masters and Johnson on Sex and Human Loving.* 1986. Little, Brown and Company.

Pallone, Nathaniel J. *Rehabilitating Criminal Psychopaths: Legislative Mandates, Clinical Quandries.* 1990. Transaction Books, New Brunswick (USA) and Oxford (U.K.).

Wolman, Benjamin B. 1989. *Dictionary of Behavioral Science, second edition.* New York: Academic Press.

INDEX